Cryonics Guidebook:
A Resource for Social Workers, Doulas, Caregivers, and Caring Others

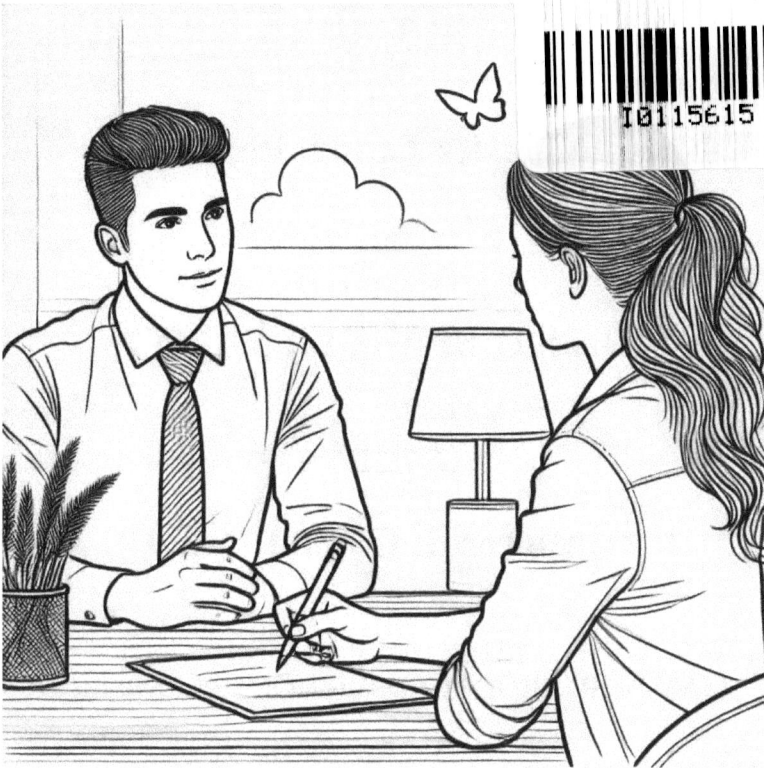

by

Charles Tandy, Ph.D.

and

Bridget Brown, L.L.B.S.W.

- 1 -

Cryonics Guidebook: A Resource for Social Workers, Doulas, Caregivers, and Caring Others

by

Charles Tandy, Ph.D.

and

Bridget Brown, L.L.B.S.W.

assisted by

Microsoft Copilot, A.I.

As a matter of feasibility, the present version of this Guidebook is oriented toward the United States.

First Edition
ISBN 978-1-934297-44-5
Printed in the United States of America
First published 2025 by Ria University Press

Preface

Brief reflections of Dr. Charles Tandy on the work as a whole.

I have been a cryonicist since the 1960s. Now living in a senior community, I asked our social worker to assist me. Bridget Brown has provided me with outstanding expertise and wise counsel.

As I briefly reflect on the completed work as a whole, these are points I think in need of emphasizing upfront:

(1) **Here are some vital points taken directly from my Advance Directive (Durable Power of Attorney for Health Care):**

Honoring someone's "last wishes" is seen as a benevolent duty in America and many other cultures. I ask that my "last wishes" be honored with an emphasis on the protocol described below.

CONCERNS:

> Standard formats may not adequately address the circumstances of the cryonics patient. *A critical task in cryonics advance planning is to clarify the patient's values, goals and wishes that the patient wants others to follow.*

> Hopefully this document will also help correct misinformation about cryonics.

> Please note that the biomedical technical papers about cryonics in the PubMed literature speak favorably of its eventual success (https://ssrn.com/abstract=2913107). Also worth noting is the Scientists' Open Letter on Cryonics (https://cryonics.org/cryonics-library/scientists-open-letter-on-cryonics).

TERMINOLOGIES:

> **Actual or Information Death** is not the same thing as Legal Death. **Actual or Information Death** is the *irreversible* loss of life. **Actual or Information Death** is the loss of *brain structures* encoding memory and personality to the extent that it's physically impossible for *any technology* to infer them, making recovery of the original person impossible by any technology, even the super-advanced technology of the future.

> **Legal Death** is NOT the same thing as Actual or Information Death. **Legal Death** is a determination of death for *legal* purposes. In the United States, there are two methods by which legal death can be pronounced: (1) **Brain Death**; and, (2) **Clinical or Cardiopulmonary Death**.

> **Brain Death**: In the mid-20th century it was observed that sometimes the brain would begin decomposing even if the heart and rest of the body remained functioning. This became called "brain death."

> **Clinical or Cardiopulmonary Death** is determined by cessation of breathing and heartbeat according to presently existing law including what resuscitation measures are *available or intended, if any*.

> **Cryonics**: If the *cryonics patient* is legally dead, then there is an established cryonics protocol to treat the patient as a sick person rather than as a corpse – for example, cryobiological vitrification (ice-free cryopreservation). Long-term cryonics care means no further deterioration. *Future developments may allow inference to healthy brain structure, and recovery of the original person to full health.*

> **Cryonics and the Two Modes of Legal Death**: (1) **Brain Death** is a disaster for cryonics. *Cryonics patients are not to be maintained on a ventilator or other life support if their prognosis for brain recovery is poor.* (2) **Clinical or Cardiopulmonary Death** is NOT NECESSARILY a disaster for cryonics. A brain

- 4 -

injured by many minutes of stopped blood circulation is a very sick brain; only much later does it become a dead brain.

MORE FROM MY ADVANCE DIRECTIVE (EXAMPLE):

The Patient (Charles E. Tandy) hereby directs everyone -- specifically including physicians, nurses, and other health care providers – to honor the concerns and terminologies mentioned above.

Ideally, the cryonics patient will at NO point undergo FREEZING but will, instead, initially undergo cooling to 34°F (1°C) and later undergo cryobiological vitrification (ice-free cryopreservation rather than freezing).

Ideally, the legal death of the patient (Charles E. Tandy) is followed INSTANTANEOUSLY by cryonics measures **that treat the patient as a person (as an ONGOING patient, not as a corpse).** If the cryonics patient is legally dead, then there is an established cryonics protocol to treat the patient as a person rather than as a corpse. This eventually involves cooling of the patient to cryogenic temperature such as via cryobiological vitrification (ice-free cryopreservation). Then the patient is placed in long-term cryonics care at cryogenic temperature (such as via liquid nitrogen). This means no further deterioration, thus the patient is waiting for future technological, medical, and rejuvenation developments. Such future developments may allow inference to healthy brain structure, and recovery of the original person to full health.

Whole Body Donor – URGENT!
Uniform Anatomical Gift Act

Do NOT Autopsy! Do NOT Embalm! Do NOT Freeze!

(2)
Two keys necessary for a good cryonic preservation are:

- Immediate pronouncement of legal death; and,
- Immediate initiation of the cryonics process.

Without these foundations, the cryonics process is compromised. Both the client and the professional social worker, doula, or caregiver must position these underpinnings at the forefront of their cryonics planning and real-life implementation. **It is NOT easy to get this right.**

(3)
Good communication is another vital point:

Effective communication is essential when discussing cryonics. This includes conversations with doctors, nurses, and other fellow professionals. The topic can be convoluted, emotional, and sometimes controversial. Whether in terms of professionals or laypersons, there seems to be a lot of misinformation out there. (One idea is to provide a free e-copy or hardcopy of this Preface or Guidebook to the professional or layperson before one's first serious conversation with them.)

The field of cryonics continues to develop. It is becoming increasingly important for those in caregiving professions—such as social workers, doulas, and other caregivers—to understand its principles and implications and the support needs of those considering this option. Not to be overlooked is that many cryonics clients are young and healthy. Also not to be overlooked is that there are about as many animals (family pets) in cryonic preservation as humans. By focusing on individualized care, collaboration, and continuous improvement, professional social workers, doulas, and caregivers can provide a valuable service that supports clients and their families throughout the cryonics process.

Abstract

The **Cryonics Guidebook** provides a valuable resource for social workers, doulas, caregivers, and others involved in end-of-life care and end-of-life-cycle care. The necessity of this guidebook arises from a growing recognition that cryonics is not merely a futuristic concept but a present reality. The guidebook provides an overview of cryonics, including scientific principles, ethical and legal issues, and alternative definitions of death. Techniques of support, advocacy, and counseling, and strategies of preparation, planning, and communication, are provided. Future advancements in cryonics and their implications are examined. For those who are young and healthy, cryonics can be incorporated into a pro healthspan extension lifestyle. The concept of "turnkey cryonics" emphasizes the importance of individualizing cryonics to each unique client and circumstance.

Keywords

1. Caregivers;
2. Counseling techniques;
3. Cryogenics;
4. Cryonics;
5. Cryopreservation;
6. Definitions of death;
7. Doulas;
8. End-of-life care / end-of-life-cycle care;
9. Healthspan extension / life extension;
10. Life on hold;
11. Social workers;
12. Turnkey cryonics;
13. VSED (voluntarily stopping eating and drinking).

Meet the Authors

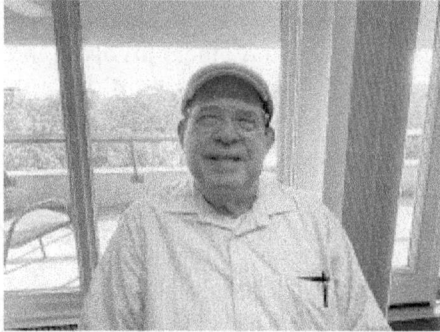

(Photo) Charles Tandy, Ph.D. (2024)

Charles Tandy now lives in a senior community. Tandy received his Ph.D. in Philosophy of Education from the University of Missouri at Columbia (USA) before becoming a Visiting Scholar in the Philosophy Department at Stanford University (USA). More at: <www.DrTandy.com> and <ssrn.com/author=2026015>. (ORCID: <https://orcid.org/0000-0003-2174-6082>).

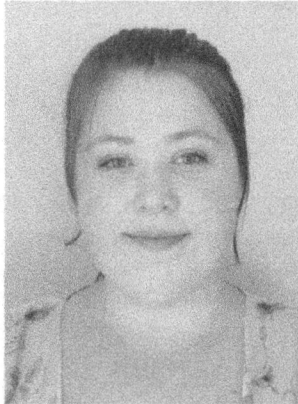

(Photo) Bridget Brown, L.L.B.S.W. (2022)

Bridget Brown is a recent graduate of Eastern Michigan University (USA): Bachelors in Social Work with a focus on the aging community. Grade: 3.7 GPA. Halle Social Justice Scholar. More at: <https://www.linkedin.com/in/bridget-carey-brown>.

Cryonics Guidebook: A Resource for Social Workers, Doulas, Caregivers, and Caring Others

—TABLE OF CONTENTS—

PART ONE: Introduction

- **SECTION 1: Purpose of the Guidebook**: Explanation of the need for a guidebook on cryonics for social workers, doulas, and caregivers.

- **SECTION 2: Overview of Cryonics**: Brief description of what cryonics is and its goals.

Section 1: Purpose of the Guidebook

Explanation of the need for a guidebook on cryonics for social workers, doulas, and caregivers.

Introduction

Cryonics, the practice of preserving individuals at extremely low temperatures with the hope of future revival, is a topic that often evokes a mix of curiosity, skepticism, and hope. As this field continues to develop, it becomes increasingly important for those in caregiving professions—such as social workers, doulas, and other caregivers—to understand its principles and implications and the support needs of those considering this option.

Why This Guidebook?

The chief aim of this guidebook is to provide a preparatory resource for social workers, doulas, caregivers, and other caring individuals who may encounter clients or patients interested in cryonics. This guidebook seeks to demystify cryonics, offering clear, factual information and practical advice to help caregivers provide informed and compassionate support.

Bridging the Knowledge Gap

Cryonics is an often misunderstood field. Many caregivers may not have had the opportunity to learn about cryonics in their formal training. This guidebook aims to bridge that knowledge gap by presenting the scientific, ethical, and quotidian (practical) aspects of cryonics in an accessible manner.

Supporting Informed Decisions

One of the key roles of caregivers is to support individuals in making informed decisions about their care. This guidebook will equip caregivers with the knowledge and tools needed to discuss cryonics with their clients or patients, helping them to understand the potential benefits and limitations, and to make decisions that align with their values and wishes.

Addressing Ethical and Emotional Concerns

Cryonics raises several ethical and emotional questions. Caregivers often find themselves navigating these multifaceted issues alongside their clients or patients. This guidebook will explore these concerns, guiding how to approach sensitive conversations and offer emotional support throughout the decision-making process.

Practical Guidance for Caregivers

In addition to providing background information, this guidebook will offer practical advice on how to support clients or patients who choose cryonics. This includes guidance on legal and logistical preparations, communication strategies, and case studies that illustrate real-life experiences and lessons learned.

A Resource for the Future

As cryonics technology and practices continue to evolve, the need for informed and compassionate caregivers will only grow. This guidebook is designed to be a living resource, one that can be updated and expanded as new information and best practices emerge.

Conclusion

By providing a thorough understanding of cryonics and its implications, this guidebook aims to empower social workers, doulas, caregivers, and other caring individuals to support their clients or patients with confidence and compassion. Whether you are new to the concept of cryonics or looking to deepen your knowledge, this guidebook is here to guide you every step of the way.

Section 2: Overview of Cryonics

Brief description of what cryonics is and its goals.

Introduction

Cryonics is a fascinating and evolving field that aims to preserve human life at extremely low temperatures with the hope of future revival. This Section provides a broad overview of cryonics, including its history, scientific principles, and current practices. Not to be overlooked is that many cryonics clients are young and healthy. Also not to be overlooked is that there are about as many animals (pets) in cryonic preservation as humans.

History and Development

The concept of cryonics was popularized in the 1960s by Robert Ettinger, often referred to as the father of cryonics. His book, *The Prospect of Immortality*, published in 1964, laid the groundwork for the modern cryonics movement. The first human to be cryonically preserved was James Bedford in 1967. Since then, the field has seen significant advancements, although it remains a niche practice.

Scientific Principles

Cryonics is based on the principle that life can be paused and potentially restarted if its basic structures can be preserved. The process involves cooling the body to subfreezing temperatures to halt biological decay. This is achieved through a process called vitrification, which uses cryoprotectants to prevent ice formation and preserve cellular structures.

1. Cryopreservation Process: The procedure plans to begin the process immediately after legal death is declared. A simplified description of the cryonics protocol is as follows: The body is chilled. Blood is replaced with cryoprotective agents to prevent ice formation. Next, the cryonics patient is gradually cooled to cryogenic temperature. Then comes long-term cryonics care. Typically this means placement in liquid nitrogen at $-196°C$.

2. Vitrification: This technique transforms biological tissues into a glass-like state, avoiding the damage caused by ice crystals. Proper cryopreservation is crucial for preserving the fine structures of the brain, which are essential for memory and personality.

Current Practices

Cryonics is currently practiced by a few specialized organizations, primarily headquartered in the United States. Founded in the 1970s in the United States, these non-profit organizations offer services ranging from whole-body preservation to neuropreservation, where only the brain is preserved. Like the cost of a car or a house, the cost of cryonics can vary considerably. (For example: How much is the client willing to pay for a bedside cryonics standby team, large or small?) In cryonics, a life insurance policy is an acceptable manner of payment.

1. Whole-Body Preservation: This involves preserving the entire body with the hope that future technology will be able to repair and revive it.

2. Neuropreservation: This focuses on preserving the brain, based on the belief that future advancements may allow for the regeneration of a new body and/or the transfer of consciousness to a different substrate.

Ethical and Legal Considerations

Cryonics raises ethical and legal questions. Ethical debates may center around the definition of death or the consent of the individual being preserved. In conformity with United States law, cryonics in the United States is only performed after a person has been declared legally dead, which varies by jurisdiction.

1. Ethical Issues: Concerns here include informed consent, the definition of death, and the potential societal impacts of cryonics.

2. Legal Status: The legal framework for cryonics varies from region to region.

Future Prospects

The future of cryonics is closely tied to scientific-technological advancements, such as in biomedical innovation, cryobiology, nanotech, quantum tech, synthetic biology, and AI. Researchers are optimistic that future technologies will enable the repair of cellular damage. Arguably, the revival of cryonically preserved individuals will become possible using future technology. However, cryonics remains an experimental field with many uncertainties.

Conclusion

Cryonics represents a bold and hopeful vision for the future, aiming to extend human life beyond the limits of current medical science. By understanding its principles, history, and current practices, caregivers can better support individuals considering this option and navigate the ethical, legal, and quotidian landscape surrounding it.

PART TWO: Understanding Cryonics

- **SECTION 3: History and Development**: A brief history of cryonics and its evolution.

- **SECTION 4: Scientific Principles**: Basic scientific concepts behind cryonics, including cryopreservation and potential revival.

Section 3: History and Development

A brief history of cryonics and its evolution.

Introduction

The journey of cryonics from a speculative idea to a developing field is a fascinating tale of scientific curiosity, technological innovation, and philosophical debate. This Section explores the history and development of cryonics, highlighting key milestones and the visionaries who have shaped its progress.

Early Concepts and Inspirations

The idea of preserving human life through freezing, low temperature, or by other means can be traced back to early science fiction literature. These imaginative works laid the groundwork for the scientific exploration of cryonics.

The Birth of Modern Cryonics

The modern cryonics movement began in earnest in the 1960s, largely due to the efforts of Robert Ettinger. Ettinger, a college teacher of physics and mathematics, published *The Prospect of Immortality* in 1964. In this seminal book, he argued that freezing individuals at the time of legal death could preserve them until future medical advancements could revive and cure them.

1. Robert Ettinger: Often called the father of cryonics, Ettinger's work inspired the formation of cryonics organizations in the 1960s and 1970s and laid the philosophical and scientific foundations for the field.

2. First Cryopreservation: The first human to be cryonically preserved was Dr. James Bedford. (As a University of California professor of psychology, he had specialized in occupational counseling.) Cryopreserved in 1967 and continuously thereafter, his body remains cryopreserved today, serving as a symbol of the early cryonics movement.

Formation of Cryonics Organizations

Following Ettinger's publication, cryonics organizations were established to promote and practice cryonics. These organizations played a crucial role in advancing the field.

The Cryonics Institute (CI), founded by Robert Ettinger in 1976, is one of the oldest and most prominent cryonics organizations. It offers whole-body cryopreservation services and has been involved in numerous research initiatives. **The Alcor Life Extension Foundation (Alcor)**, established even earlier, in 1972, is another leading cryonics organization. It is known for its rigorous scientific approach and has been at the forefront of developing advanced cryopreservation techniques.

Technological Advancements

The field of cryonics has seen significant technological advancements since its inception. Early methods of freezing often resulted in ice crystal formation, which damaged cells and tissues. The development of vitrification, a process that prevents ice formation by turning biological tissues into a glass-like state, marked a breakthrough.

The development of effective cryoprotectants has been essential for successful cryopreservation. These substances protect cells from damage during the cooling and thawing processes. Introduced in the late 20th century, vitrification uses cryoprotectants to preserve cellular structures without ice damage. This technique has improved the viability of cryopreserved tissues.

Ethical and Legal Milestones

Cryonics has also navigated a varied landscape of ethical and legal challenges. Debates over the definition of death, informed consent, and the potential societal impacts of cryonics have shaped its perception and development.

1. Ethical Debates: The ethical implications of cryonics, including issues of informed consent and the definition of death, have been debated. These discussions have influenced public perception.

2. Legal Frameworks: Historically, the legal status of cryonics in the United States is that it is legal, based on the fact that it is "not illegal." But on the "legal by being explicitly legal" side of the ledger, legal recognition of cryonics as a legitimate practice has been growing since the 1990s.

Current State and Future Directions

Today, cryonics remains an experimental field with a small but dedicated following. Ongoing research aims to improve cryopreservation techniques and explore the potential for future revival. The future of cryonics is closely tied to advancements in many fields of research, such as nanotechnology, regenerative medicine, and artificial intelligence.

1. Research and Development: Current research focuses on improving cryopreservation methods, understanding the effectiveness of alternative protocols and procedures, and developing potential revival techniques.

2. Future Prospects: The future of cryonics holds exciting possibilities for the revival of one's self and of one's friends – into a world in which indefinitely extended healthspans are the norm. Perhaps technological and biomedical advancements will transform cryonics from a speculative experimental or emergency practice into a viable option for healthspan extension, including the reversal of aging and an end to the debilities and disabilities of chronic diseases and old age.

Conclusion

The history and development of cryonics is a testament to human ingenuity and the enduring quest for healthy life extension. By understanding its past, caregivers can better appreciate the challenges and potential of cryonics, and support individuals considering this option with informed and compassionate care.

Section 4: Scientific Principles

Basic scientific concepts behind cryonics, including cryopreservation and potential revival.

Introduction

Cryonics is grounded in scientific principles that aim to preserve human life at extremely low temperatures with the hope of future revival. This Section delves into the key scientific concepts that underpin cryonics, including the processes of cryopreservation and vitrification, and the potential for future revival.

Cryopreservation Process

Cryopreservation is the process of preserving biological systems at very low temperatures to halt all biological activity and prevent decay. In cryonics, the goal is to maintain structural integrity over a (perhaps long) period until future technologies can potentially revive and repair the patient to a healthy state.

1. Initial Cooling: Immediately after legal death is declared, the body is cooled (typically using ice) to slow down metabolic processes. This is a critical step to minimize cellular damage.

2. Cryoprotectant Perfusion: Blood is replaced with cryoprotective agents, which are chemicals that protect cells from ice damage. This process, known as perfusion, helps to prevent the formation of ice crystals that can lead to cellular damage.

3. Vitrification: The body is gradually cooled to a temperature where the cryoprotectants cause the tissues to vitrify, or turn into a glass-like state. This prevents ice formation and preserves cellular structures.

4. Long-Term Care: Typically, the vitrified body is then cooled to −196°C and placed in liquid nitrogen. At this temperature, all biological processes are effectively halted, and the body can be preserved indefinitely.

Vitrification

Vitrification is a key technique in cryonics that prevents the formation of ice crystals, which can cause significant damage to cells and tissues. Instead of freezing, vitrification turns biological tissues into a glass-like state, maintaining their structural integrity.

1. Cryoprotectants: Cryoprotectants are substances used to protect biological tissues from freezing damage. They work by lowering the freezing point of water and preventing ice crystal formation.

2. Glass Transition: During vitrification, the cryoprotectants cause the water in cells to enter a glass-like state, known as the glass transition. This state preserves the fine structures of the cells without the formation of ice.

3. Advantages of Vitrification: Vitrification offers significant advantages over traditional freezing methods, including better preservation of cellular structures and reduced risk of ice damage.

Potential for Future Revival

The ultimate goal of cryonics is to revive preserved individuals in the future when medical and technological advancements have progressed sufficiently. While this remains speculative, several scientific concepts provide a basis for this hope.

1. Nanotechnology: Advances in nanotechnology could enable the repair of cellular and molecular damage caused by the cryopreservation process. Futuristic nanobots, tiny machines capable of manipulating individual molecules, could potentially restore cells to their original state.

2. Regenerative Medicine: Developments in regenerative medicine, including stem cell therapy and tissue engineering, could allow for the regeneration of damaged tissues and organs. This could be crucial for reviving cryonically preserved individuals.

3. Mind Uploading: Another speculative concept is mind uploading, where the contents of a person's brain are transferred to a digital or artificial substrate. This could offer an additional alternative path to revival, preserving the individual's consciousness and identity.

Current Research and Challenges

Cryonics is an experimental field, and many challenges remain. Ongoing research aims to address these challenges and improve the viability of cryopreservation and potential revival.

1. Cryoprotectant Toxicity: One of the major challenges is the toxicity of cryoprotectants, which can cause damage to cells. Researchers are working to develop less toxic cryoprotectants and improve perfusion techniques.

2. Ice Formation: Despite advances in vitrification, preventing ice formation remains a critical challenge. Research is focused on optimizing cooling rates and cryoprotectant formulations to minimize ice damage.

3. Revival Techniques: The development of reliable revival techniques is still in its infancy. Research in nanotechnology, regenerative medicine, and neuroscience is crucial for making revival a realistic possibility. Future biotechnological techniques may differ greatly from current techniques.

Conclusion

By understanding the scientific principles underlying cryonics, caregivers can better appreciate the potential and limitations of cryonics, and provide informed support to individuals considering this option. While many challenges remain, ongoing research and technological advancements offer hope for the future of cryonics.

PART THREE: Ethical and Legal Considerations

- **SECTION 5: Ethical Issues**: Discussion of the ethical debates surrounding cryonics, including consent and the definition of death.

- **SECTION 6: Legal Framework**: Overview of the legal status of cryonics in different regions and the implications for practitioners.

Section 5: Ethical Issues

Discussion of the ethical debates surrounding cryonics, including consent and the definition of death.

Introduction

Cryonics, with its hope of future revival, raises a host of ethical questions that are crucial for social workers, doulas, caregivers, and other caring individuals to consider. This Section explores the ethical issues surrounding cryonics, including consent, the definition of death, and the broader societal implications.

Informed Consent

One of the most fundamental ethical principles in cryonics is informed consent. Ensuring that individuals fully understand the process, arguments, and uncertainties involved in cryonics is essential.

1. Autonomy and Decision-Making: Respecting the autonomy of individuals means ensuring they have all the necessary information to make an informed decision about cryonics. This includes understanding the experimental nature of the procedure and the current limitations of the technology.

2. Capacity to Consent: Assessing an individual's capacity to consent is critical, especially in cases where cognitive impairments or terminal illnesses are involved. Caregivers must ensure that consent is given freely and without coercion.

3. Advance Directives: Encouraging individuals to document their wishes regarding cryonics in advance directives can help ensure their preferences are respected, even if they become unable to communicate them later.

Pausing Life and Defining Death

Cryonics challenges us to clarify the various possible definitions of death, as it involves preserving individuals at the point of legal death with the hope of future revival.

1. Legal Death: The distinction between legal death and actual death is crucial in cryonics. Legal death is a determination of death for legal purposes.

2. Actual Death: Death (actual death) is the irreversible loss of life. (Many meanings given to death, such as when used with a variety of adjectives, are not consistent with the meaning of actual death.) Death is the (absolutely) irreversible loss of life, making recovery of the original person impossible by any technology, even by the super-technology of the future. Many cryonicists today would define (actual) death as the loss of brain structures encoding memory and personality to an extent that it's physically impossible for any technology, no matter how super-advanced, to infer them.

3. Paused Life: The distinction in cryonics between death and legal death suggests thinking in terms of putting life on hold, the pausing of life. Thus some cryonicists will use terms like cryonic hibernation, cryonic suspension, and so on.

Ethical Debates

Cryonics is the subject of ongoing ethical debates, with arguments both for and against the practice.

1. Arguments in Favor: Proponents argue that cryonics offers a chance at life extension and the possibility of future medical advancements that could cure or reverse currently incurable conditions. They see it as an extension of the right to life and an expression of hope and optimism.

2. Arguments Against: Critics raise concerns about the experimental nature of cryonics, the potential for false hope, and the ethical implications of reviving individuals in an uncertain future. They also question the allocation of resources to cryonics when there are pressing healthcare needs in the present.

Societal Implications

The broader societal implications of cryonics are significant and warrant careful consideration.

1. Resource Allocation: The resources required for cryonics, including financial, technological, and medical resources, raise questions about their allocation. Critics argue that these resources could be better used to address current healthcare challenges.

2. Equity and Access: Currently, cryonics is not covered by Medicare or Medicaid and it is typically not offered free of charge. Cryonic preservation normally requires significant financial means comparable to buying a car or a house. (Life insurance is often proffered as payment.) At least for some, this raises ethical concerns about equity and access, and the potential for cryonics to exacerbate social inequalities.

3. Impact on Future Generations: According to some authors, the revival of cryonically preserved individuals could have profound implications for future generations. For example, ethical considerations such as the potential burden on future societies or the responsibilities of those who choose cryonics today.

Emotional and Psychological Considerations

The emotional and psychological aspects of cryonics are also important ethical considerations.

1. Hope and Expectations: Managing the hopes and expectations of individuals and their families is crucial. Caregivers must provide realistic information about the current state of cryonics and the uncertainties involved.

2. Grief and Loss: Cryonics can complicate the grieving process for families and loved ones. Caregivers should be prepared to support individuals through complex emotions and help them navigate their grief.

3. Psychological Impact of Revival: If revival becomes possible, the psychological impact on individuals who are revived after a long period of preservation must be considered. This includes potential challenges in adjusting to a future society and the loss of connections to their past life. (Note, however, that choosing cryonics is possible too for one's friends and relatives. In cryonics, family-wide decisions are not unknown, likewise pricing discounts for families.)

Conclusion

The ethical issues surrounding cryonics are multifaceted. By understanding these issues, caregivers can provide informed and compassionate support to individuals considering cryonics. Navigating the ethical landscape of cryonics suggests or requires thoughtful consideration of issues such as informed consent, the definition of death, societal implications, and the emotional and psychological impact on individuals and their families.

Section 6: Legal Framework

Overview of the legal status of cryonics in different regions
and the implications for practitioners.

Introduction

Cryonics operates within a legal landscape that varies across
different regions. Understanding the legal framework is essential
for social workers, doulas, caregivers, and other caring individuals
who counsel clients considering cryonics. This Section explores
the legal aspects of cryonics, including its status, regulatory
challenges, and key legal considerations.

Legal Status of Cryonics

Cryonics is not explicitly regulated in many jurisdictions, which
can lead to legal challenges. In the United States, there are no
federal laws specifically addressing cryonics. However, various
state laws and regulations can impact cryonics practices,
particularly those related to the declaration of death, handling of
human remains, and consumer protection.

Key Legal Considerations

Several key legal considerations are crucial for understanding and
navigating the legal landscape of cryonics.

1. Declaration of Death: Cryonics procedures typically begin
immediately after legal death is declared. The criteria for declaring
death can vary by jurisdiction, impacting the timing and legality of
cryopreservation.

2. Consent and Advance Directives: Ensuring informed consent
is a fundamental legal requirement. Advance directives and legal
documents outlining an individual's wishes regarding cryonics are
essential to ensure their preferences are respected.

3, Handling of Human Remains: Laws governing the handling, transportation, and management of human remains can affect cryonics practices. Compliance with these regulations is crucial to avoid legal complications.

4. Consumer Protection: Cryonics organizations must adhere to consumer protection laws, which may include regulations on advertising, contracts, and financial transactions. Ensuring transparency and honesty in communications is essential.

Regulatory Challenges

Cryonics faces several regulatory challenges that can impact its practice and development.

1. Lack of Specific Regulations: The absence of specific regulations for cryonics can lead to legal uncertainties and challenges. This can affect the ability of cryonics organizations to operate and provide services consistently.

2. Interdisciplinary Legal Issues: Cryonics intersects with various areas of law, including medical law, property law, and financial regulation. Navigating these interdisciplinary legal issues requires a comprehensive understanding of the relevant legal principles.

3. Legal Precedents: Legal cases and precedents can significantly influence the practice of cryonics. For example, court decisions in the U.S. and Europe have addressed issues such as the right to be cryopreserved and the enforcement of cryonics contracts.

Ethical and Legal Intersections

The ethical and legal aspects of cryonics are closely intertwined, with ethical considerations often influencing legal decisions and vice versa.

1. Ethical Debates: Ethical debates about the definition of death, informed consent, and the potential societal impacts of cryonics can shape legal frameworks and regulatory approaches.

2. Legal Protections: Legal protections for individuals choosing cryonics, such as the right to make decisions about their own bodies and the enforcement of advance directives, are essential for ensuring ethical practices.

Future Directions

The legal landscape of cryonics is likely to evolve as the field develops and as societal attitudes towards healthspan extension and cryonic preservation mature.

1. Advocacy and Legislation: Successful advocacy efforts aimed at establishing clearer legal frameworks and protections for cryonics would help address current regulatory challenges. This may include lobbying for or against specific legislation and raising public awareness about cryonics. But advocacy efforts, if any, should be pursued cautiously with political backlash in mind. Historically important for cryonics, as for numerous other activities, is the dictum: legal because it is "not illegal."

2. International Collaboration: Arguably, international collaboration among cryonics organizations, legal experts, and policymakers can help harmonize regulations and promote best practices globally.

3. Ongoing Research: Continued research into the legal and ethical aspects of cryonics is essential for addressing emerging issues and ensuring that the practice evolves in a responsible, ethical manner.

Conclusion

Understanding the legal framework of cryonics is crucial for caregivers supporting individuals considering this option. By navigating the legal landscape, caregivers can help ensure that their clients' wishes are respected and that cryonics practices are conducted ethically and legally. As the field of cryonics continues to evolve, staying informed about legal developments and advocacy efforts will be essential for supporting informed and compassionate care.

PART FOUR: The Role of Social Workers

- **SECTION 7: Support and Advocacy**: How social workers can support individuals and families considering cryonics.

- **SECTION 8: Counseling Techniques**: Effective counseling methods for discussing cryonics with clients.

Section 7: Support and Advocacy

How social workers can support individuals and families considering cryonics.

Introduction

Supporting individuals and families considering cryonics requires a compassionate and informed approach. Social workers, doulas, caregivers, and other caring individuals play a crucial role in providing emotional support, practical assistance, and advocacy. This Section explores how caregivers can effectively support and advocate for those interested in cryonics.

Understanding the Client's Perspective

To provide effective support, it is essential to understand the motivations, hopes, and concerns of individuals considering cryonics.

1. Listening and Empathy: Active listening and empathy are fundamental. Take the time to understand the individual's reasons for choosing cryonics, their hopes for the future, and any fears or uncertainties they may have.

2. Respecting Autonomy: Respect the individual's autonomy and their right to make decisions about their own body and future. Ensure that they feel heard and validated in their choices.

Providing Emotional Support

Cryonics can evoke a range of emotions, from hope and optimism to fear and uncertainty. Providing emotional support is a key aspect of caregiving.

1. Creating a Safe Space: Create a safe and non-judgmental space where individuals can express their feelings and concerns. Encourage open and honest communication.

2. Addressing Fears and Concerns: Help individuals explore and address any fears or concerns they may have about cryonics. Provide accurate information and reassurance where possible.

3. Supporting Families: Families may also have strong emotions and concerns about cryonics. Offer support to family members, helping them understand the process and navigate their own feelings.

Practical Assistance

Providing practical assistance can help individuals and families navigate the logistical and legal aspects of cryonics.

1. Advance Directives and Legal Documents: Assist individuals in preparing advance directives and other legal documents that outline their wishes regarding cryonics. Ensure that these documents are clear and legally binding.

2. Coordination with Cryonics Organizations: Help individuals coordinate with cryonics organizations, including arranging for membership, contracts, and financial planning.

3. End-of-Life Planning: Support individuals in planning for end-of-life care and end-of-life-cycle care, including the transition to cryopreservation. This may involve coordinating with healthcare providers, hospice care, and cryonics teams.

Advocacy and Education

Advocacy and education are essential for promoting understanding and acceptance of cryonics within the broader community.

1. Raising Awareness: Raise awareness about cryonics through community education and outreach. Provide accurate information to dispel myths and misconceptions.

2. Advocating for Legal Protections: Advocate for legal protections and clear regulations for cryonics. This may involve working with policymakers, legal experts, and cryonics organizations to promote supportive legislation.

3. Supporting Research and Development: Advocate for continued research and development in cryonics and related fields. Support efforts to improve cryopreservation techniques and explore potential revival methods.

Case Studies and Personal Stories

Sharing case studies and personal stories can provide valuable insights and lessons for caregivers.

1. Real-Life Examples: Include case studies of individuals who have chosen cryonics and the experiences of their caregivers. Highlight the challenges and successes they encountered.

2. Lessons Learned: Discuss the lessons learned from these case studies, including best practices for providing support and advocacy.

Building a Support Network

Building a support network can enhance the care and advocacy provided to individuals considering cryonics.

1. **Collaboration with Professionals**: Collaborate with other professionals, including healthcare providers, legal experts, and

cryonics organizations. This multidisciplinary approach can provide comprehensive support.
2. **Peer Support Groups**: Encourage the formation of peer support groups where individuals and families can share their experiences and support each other.
3. **Continuing Education**: Stay informed about the latest developments in cryonics and related fields. Participate in continuing education opportunities to enhance your knowledge and skills.

Conclusion

Supporting and advocating for individuals considering cryonics requires a compassionate, informed, and proactive approach. By understanding their perspectives, providing emotional and practical support, and advocating for their rights, caregivers can help individuals navigate the multifarious journey of cryonics with confidence and dignity. Building a strong support network and staying informed about the latest developments will ensure that caregivers are well-equipped to provide the best possible care.

Section 8: Counseling Techniques

Effective counseling methods for discussing cryonics with clients.

Introduction

Counseling individuals and families considering cryonics requires a unique set of skills and approaches. This Section provides practical counseling techniques tailored to the specific needs and concerns of those exploring cryonics. By employing these techniques, social workers, doulas, caregivers, and other caring individuals can offer effective support and guidance.

Building Trust and Rapport

Establishing a trusting relationship is the foundation of effective counseling.

1. Active Listening: Practice active listening by giving your full attention, nodding, and providing verbal affirmations. This helps clients feel heard and understood.

2. Empathy and Compassion: Show empathy and compassion by acknowledging the client's feelings and experiences. Use phrases like, "I understand this is a difficult decision for you."

3. Non-Judgmental Attitude: Maintain a non-judgmental attitude, respecting the client's beliefs and choices regarding cryonics.

Providing Information and Education

Clients need accurate and comprehensive information to make informed decisions about cryonics.

1. Clear and Concise Information: Provide clear and concise information about the cryonics process, including its benefits, risks, and uncertainties. Use simple language and avoid technical jargon.

2. Educational Materials: Offer educational materials, such as brochures, articles, and videos, to help clients understand cryonics better. Ensure these materials are from reputable sources.

3. Answering Questions: Be prepared to answer questions and address concerns. Encourage clients to ask questions and provide honest, evidence-informed responses.

Exploring Motivations and Concerns

Understanding the client's motivations and concerns is crucial for providing personalized support.

1. Open-Ended Questions: Use open-ended questions to explore the client's reasons for considering cryonics. For example, "What interests you most about cryonics?" or "What concerns do you have about the process?"

2. Reflective Listening: Reflect back what the client says to ensure understanding and validate their feelings. For example, "It sounds like you're hopeful about future medical advancements."

3. Addressing Fears: Help clients articulate and address their fears and concerns. Provide reassurance and support, and offer information to alleviate any misconceptions.

Facilitating Decision-Making

Support clients in making informed and autonomous decisions about cryonics.

1. Decision-Making Frameworks: Introduce decision-making frameworks, such as pros and cons lists or decision matrices, to help clients weigh their options.

2. Encouraging Autonomy: Encourage clients to make decisions that align with their values and beliefs. Reinforce that the choice is ultimately theirs to make.

3. Supportive Environment: Create a supportive environment where clients feel comfortable discussing their thoughts and feelings without pressure or judgment.

Supporting Families and Loved Ones

Families and loved ones may also need support as they navigate the decision-making process.

1. Family Counseling Sessions: Offer family counseling sessions to address the concerns and emotions of family members. Facilitate open and respectful communication.

2. Mediating Conflicts: Mediate conflicts that may arise within families regarding the decision to pursue cryonics. Help family members understand and respect each other's perspectives.

3. Providing Resources: Provide resources and information to family members to help them understand cryonics and support their loved one's decision.

Ethical Considerations in Counseling

Ethical considerations are paramount in counseling clients about cryonics.

1. Informed Consent: Ensure that clients fully understand the cryonics process and its implications before making a decision. Obtain informed consent in writing.

2. Confidentiality: Maintain confidentiality and respect the privacy of clients and their families. Ensure that all discussions and decisions are kept confidential.

3. Professional Boundaries: Maintain professional boundaries and avoid imposing personal beliefs or biases on clients. Focus on providing unbiased support and information.

Case Studies and Role-Playing

Using case studies and role-playing can enhance counseling skills and prepare for real-life scenarios.

1. Case Studies: Review case studies of individuals who have chosen cryonics and the counseling techniques used to support them. Discuss the outcomes and lessons learned.

2. Role-Playing Exercises: Engage in role-playing exercises with colleagues to practice counseling techniques. Simulate different scenarios and receive feedback to improve skills.

Conclusion

Effective counseling for individuals considering cryonics requires a combination of empathy, knowledge, and practical skills. By building trust, providing accurate information, exploring motivations and concerns, facilitating decision-making, supporting families, and adhering to ethical standards, caregivers can offer valuable support to those navigating the multifaceted journey of cryonics. Continuous learning and practice will ensure that caregivers are well-equipped to provide the best possible care.

- **SECTION 9: End-of-Life-Cycle Care**: How doulas can integrate cryonics into their end-of-life care practices.

- **SECTION 10: Emotional Support**: Providing emotional support to clients and families during the cryonics process.

Section 9: End-of-Life-Cycle Care

How doulas can integrate cryonics into their
end-of-life care practices.

Introduction

End-of-life care is a deeply personal, and potentially difficult, journey — both for the cryonics client facing the end of their current life cycle and for their loved ones. Doulas, who provide emotional, spiritual, and practical support during this time, play a crucial role in ensuring a dignified and compassionate end-of-life-cycle experience. With the growing interest in cryonics, doulas are now encountering new challenges and opportunities in their practice. Not to be overlooked is that many cryonics clients are young and healthy. Also not to be overlooked is that there are about as many animals (pets) in cryonic preservation as humans. This Section explores how doulas can integrate cryonics into their end-of-life-cycle care practices, offering guidance on navigating this unique and evolving field.

Understanding Cryonics

Cryonics is the process of preserving individuals at extremely low temperatures with the hope that future medical advancements will allow for their revival and treatment of currently incurable conditions. While cryonics remains a controversial and largely experimental practice, it is gaining traction among those who wish to explore all possible avenues for extending healthspan.

The Role of Doulas in Cryonics

Arguably, at an early age, one should incorporate cryonics into a general lifestyle program to optimize one's healthspan. Doulas can play a pivotal role in supporting clients who choose cryonics as part of their end-of-life-cycle or healthspan extension plan. This involves understanding the cryonics process, addressing emotional and ethical concerns, and providing practical assistance.

1. Education and Awareness: Doulas should educate themselves about the basics of cryonics, including the scientific principles, legal considerations, and the steps involved in the cryopreservation process. This knowledge will enable doulas to answer questions and provide accurate information to clients and their families.

2. Emotional Support: Choosing cryonics can be an emotionally charged decision. Doulas can offer a non-judgmental space for clients to express their hopes, fears, and uncertainties. Active listening, empathy, and validation are key components of this support.

3. Ethical Considerations: Doulas must navigate the ethical issues associated with cryonics. This includes respecting the client's autonomy and wishes while also considering the potential impact on family members and loved ones. Open and honest communication is essential to address any ethical dilemmas that may arise.

4. Practical Assistance: Doulas can assist with the logistical aspects of cryonics, such as coordinating with cryonics organizations, ensuring legal documentation is in place, and helping families understand the procedural steps. This practical support can alleviate some of the stress and confusion associated with the cryonics process.

Integrating Cryonics into End-of-Life Care

To effectively integrate cryonics into their practice, doulas should consider the following strategies:

1. Building a Knowledge Base: Stay informed about the latest developments in cryonics by attending workshops, reading relevant literature, and connecting with cryonics organizations. This ongoing education will enhance your ability to support clients effectively.

2. Creating a Supportive Network: Establish relationships with professionals in the cryonics field, such as cryonics organizations, legal experts, and healthcare providers. A strong network can provide valuable resources and support for both doulas and their clients.

3. Developing Communication Skills: Effective communication is crucial when discussing cryonics with clients and their families. Doulas should practice clear, compassionate, and non-technical communication to ensure that everyone involved understands the process and implications of cryonics.

4. Personal Reflection and Self-Care: Working with clients who choose cryonics can be emotionally demanding. Doulas should engage in regular self-reflection and self-care practices to maintain their well-being and provide the best possible support to their clients.

Case Study: Supporting a Client through Cryonics

To illustrate the role of doulas in cryonics, consider the following (fictional) case study related to healthspan extension:

Case Study: Jane, a 40-year-old woman who recently recovered from breast cancer, decides to pursue whether she wants to incorporate cryonics into a general lifestyle program to optimize her healthspan. Her doula, Sarah, supports her through the decision-making process, providing information about cryonics and addressing Jane's emotional concerns. Jane decides to make cryonics a part of her wellness program and chooses Sarah to help provide a dependable turnkey approach to cryonics. Sarah coordinates with a cryonics organization to ensure all legal and logistical arrangements are in place. Throughout the process,

Sarah offers compassionate support to Jane and her family, helping them navigate the emotional and practical challenges of cryonics.

Conclusion

Integrating cryonics into end-of-life care presents unique challenges and opportunities for doulas. Upon legal death, the (pro healthspan extension) client becomes a cryonics patient instead of a corpse. Doulas, by educating themselves, providing emotional and practical support, and navigating ethical considerations, can play a vital role in supporting clients who choose cryonics. This Section has outlined the key aspects of this integration, offering guidance for doulas to enhance their practice and provide compassionate care to those exploring cryonics as an end-of-life-cycle or healthspan extension option.

Section 10: Emotional Support

Providing emotional support to clients and families during the cryonics process.

Introduction

The decision to pursue cryonics can be a deeply emotional journey for individuals and their families. As a social worker, doula, caregiver, or caring other, your role in providing emotional support is crucial. This Section explores the various ways you can offer compassionate and effective emotional support to clients and their families during the cryonics process.

Understanding the Emotional Landscape

Cryonics, the preservation of individuals at extremely low temperatures with the hope of future revival, is a choice that often comes with a mix of hope, fear, uncertainty, and even skepticism. Understanding the emotional landscape of clients and their families is the first step in providing meaningful support.

1. Hope and Optimism: Many individuals who choose cryonics do so with the hope of future medical advancements. This optimism can be a source of strength but may also lead to unrealistic expectations.

2. Fear and Anxiety: The unknown aspects of cryonics can generate fear and anxiety. Clients may worry about the process, the future, and the impact on their loved ones.

3. Grief and Loss: Even with the hope of future revival, the immediate reality is that the individual is facing the end of their current life cycle. This can lead to feelings of grief and loss for both the individual and their family.

4. Skepticism and Doubt: Cryonics is still a controversial and experimental practice. Clients and their families may experience doubt and skepticism, both from within and from others.

Providing Emotional Support

1. Active Listening: One of the most powerful tools you have is the ability to listen. Provide a safe and non-judgmental space for clients and their families to express their thoughts and feelings. Active listening involves being fully present, acknowledging their emotions, and validating their experiences.

2. Empathy and Compassion: Show empathy and compassion by putting yourself in their shoes. Understand their fears, hopes, and concerns. Use empathetic language and offer reassurance without making unrealistic promises.

3. Education and Information: Providing clear and accurate information about the cryonics process can help alleviate some fears and uncertainties. Be prepared to answer questions and address misconceptions. Ensure that clients and their families have access to reliable resources.

4. Emotional Validation: Validate the emotions of clients and their families. Let them know that it is okay to feel a range of emotions, from hope to fear to grief. Emotional validation helps individuals feel understood and supported.

5. Support Networks: Encourage clients and their families to build and rely on support networks. This can include friends, family, support groups, and professional counselors. A strong support network can provide additional emotional and practical assistance.

6. Mindfulness and Stress Reduction: Introduce mindfulness and stress reduction techniques to help manage anxiety and emotional distress. Practices such as deep breathing, meditation, and guided imagery can be beneficial.

7. Ethical Considerations: Be mindful of the ethical considerations involved in supporting clients who choose cryonics. Respect their autonomy and decisions while also considering the emotional impact on their families. Open and honest communication is key.

A Fictional Case Study: Emotional Support in Action

Case Study: John, a 65-year-old man with a terminal illness, decides to pursue cryonics as emergency medicine and the potential for healthspan extension. His family is supportive but also experiences a range of emotions, including hope, fear, and skepticism. His doula, Maria, provides emotional support by actively listening to John's concerns, offering empathetic reassurance, and educating the family about the cryonics process. Maria also facilitates family meetings to discuss their feelings and encourages them to seek additional support from a social worker or counselor. Through her compassionate support, Maria helps John and his family navigate an emotional journey.

Conclusion

Providing emotional support to clients and their families during the cryonics process is a multifaceted and deeply rewarding aspect of caregiving. By understanding the emotional landscape, offering empathetic and compassionate support, and addressing ethical considerations, you can help individuals and their loved ones navigate this unique and challenging journey. Your role as a social worker, doula, caregiver, or caring other is invaluable in ensuring that clients feel supported, understood, and cared for during this profound experience.

PART SIX: Practical Considerations for Caregivers

- **SECTION 11: Preparation and Planning**: Steps to prepare for cryopreservation, including legal and logistical arrangements.

- **SECTION 12: Communication Strategies**: Best practices for communicating with clients and families about cryonics.

Section 11: Preparation and Planning

Steps to prepare for cryopreservation, including legal and logistical arrangements.

Introduction

Preparation and planning are critical components of the cryonics process. For social workers, doulas, caregivers, and caring others, understanding the necessary steps and considerations can ensure a smooth and respectful transition to long term care as a cryonics patient instead of becoming a corpse. This Section outlines the essential legal and logistical arrangements required to prepare for cryopreservation.

Understanding Cryonic Preservation

Cryonic preservation involves preserving individuals at extremely low temperatures with the hope that future medical advancements will allow for their revival and treatment. This process requires meticulous planning and coordination to ensure that all legal, medical, and logistical aspects are addressed.

Legal Considerations

1. Advance Directives: Clients should have clear advance directives that outline their wishes regarding cryopreservation. This includes a living will and durable power of attorney for healthcare, specifying their desire for cryonics.

2. Legal Documentation: Ensure all necessary legal documents are completed and filed. This includes contracts with cryonics organizations, consent forms, and any other legal agreements required for the process.

3. Next of Kin and Executor: Designate a next of kin and an executor who are aware of and support the client's cryonics wishes. They will play a crucial role in ensuring that the client's wishes are respected and carried out.

4. Legal Counsel: It is advisable to consult with legal counsel experienced in cryonics to navigate any potential legal challenges and ensure all documentation is legally sound.

Logistical Arrangements

1. Cryonics Organization: Choose a reputable cryonics organization and establish a contract. This organization will offer set options for the client to choose from regarding the cryopreservation process, such as transportation, long term care, and future revival efforts.

2. Funding: Secure funding for the cryopreservation process. This can include life insurance policies, trusts, or other financial arrangements to cover the costs associated with cryonics.

3. Medical Coordination: Coordinate with medical professionals to ensure a seamless transition from end-of-life-cycle care to cryopreservation (and thus the potential possibility of healthspan extension). This includes informing healthcare providers of the client's wishes and ensuring they are prepared to cooperate with the cryonics organization.

4. Emergency Response Plan: Develop an emergency response plan that outlines the steps to be taken immediately after the client's legal death. This plan should include items like contact information for the cryonics organization, transportation arrangements, and any necessary medical procedures.

Practical Steps for Caregivers

1. Education and Training: Educate yourself about the cryonics process, including the scientific principles, legal requirements, and logistical steps. Training programs and workshops can provide valuable knowledge and skills.

2. Communication: Maintain open and honest communication with the client and their family. Ensure they understand the process, the legal and logistical requirements, and the potential challenges.

3. Support Networks: Build a network of professionals, including legal experts, medical providers, and cryonics organization representatives. This network can provide support and resources throughout the preparation and planning process.

4. Documentation and Record Keeping: Keep detailed records of all legal and logistical arrangements. This includes copies of legal documents, contracts, communication logs, and any other relevant information.

Fictional Case Study: Preparing for Cryopreservation

Case Study: Emily is a 60-year-old woman. After many tests they are unable to diagnose her painful illness or whether her condition is life threatening. Her social worker, Tom, serves as her counselor in this uncertain, emotional situation. Emily, with Tom's help, decides to explore cryonics and soon thereafter decides to pursue cryopreservation. Her social worker, Tom, further assists her in preparing for the cryonics process. Tom helps Emily establish a contract with a cryonics organization, secure funding through a life insurance policy, and complete her advance directives and legal documentation. He coordinates with Emily's healthcare providers to ensure they are aware of her wishes and develops an emergency response plan. Throughout the process, Tom maintains open communication with Emily and her family, providing support and guidance.

Conclusion

Preparation and planning are essential for a successful cryopreservation process. By understanding the legal and logistical requirements, social workers, doulas, caregivers, and caring others can provide invaluable support to clients choosing cryonics. This Section has outlined the key steps and considerations, offering a roadmap for ensuring a smooth and respectful transition to long term care as a cryonics patient instead of becoming a corpse.

Section 12: Communication Strategies

Best practices for communicating with clients
and families about cryonics.

Introduction

Effective communication is essential when discussing cryonics with clients and their families. The topic can be convoluted, emotional, and sometimes controversial. As social workers, doulas, caregivers, and caring others, it is crucial to approach these conversations with sensitivity, clarity, and empathy. This Section outlines best practices for communicating about cryonics, ensuring that clients and their families feel informed, supported, and respected.

Understanding the Communication Challenges

Cryonics involves scientific, ethical, and emotional dimensions that can make communication challenging. Clients and their families may have varying levels of understanding, differing opinions, and strong emotions about the subject. Recognizing these challenges is the first step in developing effective communication strategies.

1. Density of Information: Cryonics involves scientific concepts that may be difficult for some clients and families to understand. Simplifying and clearly explaining these concepts is essential.

2. Emotional Reactions: The idea of cryonics can evoke a range of emotions, from hope and curiosity to fear and skepticism. Being prepared to address these emotions with empathy is crucial.

3. Ethical and Cultural Considerations: Different individuals may have varying ethical and cultural perspectives on cryonics. Respecting these perspectives while empathetically providing accurate information is important.

Best Practices for Communication

1. Active Listening: Start by listening to the client and their family. Understand their concerns, questions, and emotions. Active listening involves being fully present, showing empathy, and validating their feelings.

2. Clear and Simple Language: Use clear and simple language when explaining cryonics. Avoid technical jargon and break down complex concepts into understandable terms. Visual aids and analogies can be helpful.

3. Provide Accurate Information: Ensure that the information you provide is accurate and up-to-date. Be honest about the current state of cryonics technology, its experimental nature, and the uncertainties involved.

4. Addressing Emotions: Acknowledge and address the emotions that arise during the conversation. Offer reassurance and support, and provide a safe space for clients and families to express their feelings.

5. Respecting Perspectives: Respect the ethical and cultural perspectives of clients and their families. Be open to discussing their beliefs and values, and avoid imposing your own views.

6. Encouraging Questions: Encourage clients and their families to ask questions. Answer them patiently and thoroughly, and be honest if you do not know the answer. Offer to find additional information if needed.

7. Building Trust: Building trust is essential for effective communication. Be transparent, reliable, and consistent in your interactions. Trust can help clients and families feel more comfortable discussing cryonics.

8. Providing Resources: Offer resources for further reading and support. This can include brochures, websites, and contact information for cryonics organizations. Providing resources empowers clients and families to make informed decisions.

Communication Strategies in Practice

1. Initial Conversations: When first introducing the topic of cryonics, start with a general overview. Explain what cryonics is, why some people choose it, and the basic process involved. Gauge the client's and family's initial reactions and address any immediate concerns.

2. Detailed Discussions: For clients and families who express interest in cryonics, provide more detailed information. Discuss the scientific principles, legal requirements, and logistical steps involved. Be prepared to revisit and clarify information as needed.

3. Emotional Support: Throughout the communication process, offer emotional support. Validate the client's and family's feelings, provide reassurance, and offer resources for additional emotional support, such as counseling or support groups.

4. Ongoing Communication: Maintain ongoing communication with the client and their family. Keep them informed about any updates or changes in the cryonics process. Regular check-ins can help address any new questions or concerns that arise.

Fictional Case Study: Effective Communication in Cryonics

Case Study: Mark, a 28-year-old man with a terminal illness, is considering cryonics. His caregiver, Lisa, begins by listening to Mark's thoughts and concerns about cryonics. She provides a clear and simple explanation of the process, using visual aids to help Mark understand. Lisa addresses Mark's emotions, offering reassurance and validating his feelings. She respects Mark's ethical perspectives and encourages him to ask questions. Throughout the process, Lisa builds trust by being transparent and reliable. She provides resources for further reading and maintains ongoing communication with Mark and his family.

Conclusion

Effective communication is the cornerstone of supporting clients and their families in the cryonics process. By listening actively, using clear language, addressing emotions, respecting perspectives, and building trust, social workers, doulas, caregivers, and caring others can ensure that clients feel informed and supported. This Section has outlined best practices and strategies for communicating about cryonics, helping you navigate these important and sensitive conversations with confidence and compassion.

PART SEVEN: Case Studies and Personal Stories

- **SECTION 13: Real-Life Examples**: Case studies of individuals who have chosen cryonics and the experiences of their caregivers.

- **SECTION 14: Lessons Learned**: Insights and lessons from these case studies.

Section 13: Real-Life Examples

Case studies of individuals who have chosen cryonics and the experiences of their caregivers.

Introduction

Real-life examples and case studies provide valuable insights into the practical and emotional aspects of cryonics. By examining the experiences of individuals who have chosen cryonics and the caregivers who supported them, we can better understand the challenges and rewards of this unique end-of-life-cycle, pro healthspan extension option. This Section presents several case studies that highlight the diverse experiences and lessons learned from those involved in the cryonics process.

Special Note from the Authors of This Guidebook

We hope to offer real-life examples in future versions of this Guidebook. In the meantime, the AI known as Microsoft Copilot has provided us with some fictional accounts of "real-life."

Case Study 1: Jane's Journey with Cryonics

Background: Jane, a 70-year-old woman diagnosed with a terminal illness, decided to pursue cryonics as a way to potentially extend her life. Her decision was driven by a strong belief in future medical advancements and a desire to explore all possible options.

Caregiver's Role: Jane's doula, Sarah, played a crucial role in supporting her through the cryonics process. Sarah provided emotional support, helped Jane understand the scientific and logistical aspects of cryonics, and coordinated with the cryonics organization.

Challenges: One of the main challenges was addressing the skepticism and concerns of Jane's family. Sarah facilitated open discussions, provided educational resources, and ensured that Jane's wishes were respected.

Outcome: Jane's cryopreservation was successfully completed. Her family, initially hesitant, came to appreciate the thorough planning and compassionate support provided by Sarah. This experience highlighted the importance of clear communication and emotional support in the cryonics process.

Case Study 2: Mark's Decision for Cryonics

Background: Mark, a 65-year-old man with a progressive neurological disorder, chose cryonics as a way to preserve his brain and potentially benefit from future treatments. Mark's decision was influenced by his background in science and his hope for future medical breakthroughs.

Caregiver's Role: Mark's social worker, Lisa, assisted him in navigating the legal and logistical aspects of cryonics. Lisa helped Mark complete the necessary legal documentation, secure funding, and establish a contract with a cryonics organization.

Challenges: Mark faced emotional challenges, including fear and uncertainty about the future. Lisa provided ongoing emotional support, encouraged Mark to express his feelings, and connected him with a support group for individuals considering cryonics.

Outcome: Mark's cryopreservation was carried out smoothly. The support and guidance provided by Lisa were instrumental in helping Mark and his family feel prepared and at peace with his decision. This case study underscores the importance of comprehensive preparation and emotional support.

Case Study 3: Emily's Cryonics Experience

Background: Emily, a 72-year-old woman with terminal cancer, decided to pursue cryonics after extensive research and discussions with her family. Emily's decision was motivated by her desire to explore all possible avenues for extending her life.

Caregiver's Role: Emily's caregiver, Tom, played a key role in supporting her through the cryonics process. Tom helped Emily understand the scientific principles, coordinated with medical professionals, and ensured that all legal and logistical arrangements were in place.

Challenges: Emily's family had mixed feelings about cryonics, with some members expressing skepticism. Tom facilitated family meetings to discuss their concerns, provided educational resources, and ensured that Emily's wishes were honored.

Outcome: Emily's cryopreservation was completed successfully. The support provided by Tom helped Emily and her family navigate the emotional and practical challenges of the cryonics process. This case study highlights the importance of family involvement and open communication.

Lessons Learned

1. Importance of Communication: Clear and open communication is essential in the cryonics process. Caregivers should facilitate discussions, provide accurate information, and address any concerns or misconceptions.

2. Emotional Support: Providing emotional support is crucial for both the individual choosing cryonics and their family. Caregivers should offer empathy, validation, and reassurance throughout the process.

3. Comprehensive Preparation: Thorough preparation, including legal and logistical arrangements, is key to a successful cryopreservation. Caregivers should assist with advance directives, legal documentation, and coordination with cryonics organizations.

4. Respecting Wishes: Respecting the individual's wishes and ensuring that their decisions are honored is fundamental.

Caregivers should advocate for the client's autonomy and support their choices.

Conclusion

Real-life examples and case studies provide valuable insights into the cryonics process and the experiences of those involved. By examining these stories, social workers, doulas, caregivers, and caring others can better understand the challenges and rewards of supporting individuals who choose cryonics. This Section has highlighted the importance of communication, emotional support, comprehensive preparation, and respecting the wishes of clients, offering valuable lessons for those involved in the cryonics adventure.

Section 14: Lessons Learned

Insights and lessons from these case studies.

Introduction

The journey of integrating cryonics into end-of-life care is filled with unique challenges and profound insights. (Many who have chosen cryonics, both young and old, are folks in good health. Some of them view cryonics as a necessary part of their pro healthspan extension lifestyle.) By reflecting on real-life examples or case studies, we can extract valuable lessons that enhance our understanding and improve our practices. Given the aforementioned context, this Section seeks to distill the key lessons learned from the experiences of individuals who have chosen cryonics and the caregivers who supported them.

Lesson 1: The Importance of Clear Communication

Effective communication is the cornerstone of successful cryonics planning and support. Clear, honest, and compassionate communication helps build trust, alleviate fears, and ensure that everyone involved understands the process.

1. Practice Active Listening: Always listen to the client's and family's concerns, questions, and emotions. This helps in addressing their needs more effectively.

2. Simplify Complex Information: Use simple language and visual aids to explain the scientific and logistical aspects of cryonics. Avoid jargon and ensure that the information is accessible.

3. Encourage Open Dialogue: Foster an environment where clients and families feel comfortable expressing their thoughts and concerns. Open dialogue helps in addressing any misconceptions and building consensus.

Lesson 2: Providing Emotional Support

Emotional support is crucial for clients and their families as they navigate the cryonics process. Recognizing and addressing the emotional landscape can make a significant difference in their experience.

1. Validate Emotions: Acknowledge and validate the range of emotions that clients and families may experience, from hope and optimism to fear and skepticism.

2. Offer Empathy and Compassion: Show empathy and compassion in all interactions. This helps in building a supportive and trusting relationship.

3. Connect to Support Networks: Encourage clients and families to connect with support groups, counselors, or other resources that can provide additional emotional support.

Lesson 3: Comprehensive Preparation and Planning

Thorough preparation and planning are essential for a smooth cryonics process. This involves addressing legal, logistical, and practical considerations well in advance.

1. Legal Documentation: Ensure that all necessary legal documents, such as advance directives and contracts with cryonics organizations, are completed and filed.

2. Logistical Arrangements: Coordinate with medical professionals, cryonics organizations, and other relevant parties to ensure that all logistical aspects are addressed.

3. Emergency Response Plan: Develop a detailed emergency response plan that outlines the steps to be taken immediately after the client's legal death.

Lesson 4: Respecting Client Autonomy

Respecting the client's autonomy and wishes is fundamental in the cryonics process. Caregivers should advocate for the client's decisions and ensure that their choices are honored.

1. Support Informed Decisions: Provide clients with all the necessary information to make informed decisions about cryonics. Respect their choices, even if they differ from your own views.

2. Advocate for the Client: Act as an advocate for the client's wishes, ensuring that their decisions are respected by family members, medical professionals, and cryonics organizations.

3. Ethical Considerations: Navigate ethical considerations with sensitivity and respect. Ensure that the client's autonomy is upheld while also considering the impact on their loved ones.

Lesson 5: Building Trust and Relationships

Building trust and strong relationships with clients and their families is essential for effective support. Trust fosters open communication and collaboration, making the cryonics process smoother and more positive.

1. Be Transparent and Reliable: Maintain transparency in all interactions and be reliable in fulfilling your commitments. This helps in building trust and credibility.

2. Foster Collaboration: Work collaboratively with clients, families, and other professionals involved in the cryonics process. Collaboration ensures that all aspects are addressed comprehensively.

3. Continuous Support: Provide continuous support throughout the cryonics journey, from initial discussions to the completion of the cryopreservation process. Regular check-ins and follow-ups help in addressing any new concerns or questions.

Conclusion

The experiences of individuals who have chosen cryonics and the caregivers who supported them offer valuable lessons for social workers, doulas, caregivers, and caring others. By focusing on clear communication, emotional support, comprehensive preparation, respecting client autonomy, and building trust, caregivers can enhance their practice and provide compassionate and effective support to those exploring cryonics. This Section has highlighted the key insights and lessons learned, offering a roadmap for navigating the unique challenges and opportunities of the cryonics process.

PART EIGHT: Future Directions

- **SECTION 15: Advancements in Cryonics**: Potential future developments in cryonics technology and practice.

- **SECTION 16: Implications for Caregivers**: How these advancements might impact the roles of social workers, doulas, and caregivers.

Section 15: Advancements in Cryonics

Potential future developments in cryonics technology and practice.

Introduction

Cryonics, the practice of preserving individuals at extremely low temperatures with the hope of future revival, is a field that continues to evolve. Technological advancements and scientific research are driving progress, offering new possibilities and improving existing methods. This Section explores the potential future developments in cryonics technology and practice, providing insights into how these advancements might shape the field and impact caregivers.

Potential Future Developments

1. Improved Cryoprotectants: Research is ongoing to develop more effective cryoprotectants that minimize toxicity and better protect cells during the cool-down process. Advances in cryoprotectant solutions could significantly improve the preservation quality and reduce potential damage.

2. Nanotechnology: Nanotechnology holds promise for cryonics, particularly in the areas of repair and revival. Future nanobots could potentially repair cellular damage at the molecular level, making the revival process more feasible. This technology could also enhance the precision of cryoprotectant delivery and distribution.

3. Organ and Tissue Preservation: Advances in organ and tissue preservation techniques could benefit cryonics. Improved methods for preserving organs at low temperatures could be applied to whole-body preservation and neuro-preservation, enhancing the overall viability of cryopreserved individuals.

4. Revival Techniques: While revival remains a theoretical possibility, advancements in medical technology and regenerative medicine could bring it closer to reality. Techniques such as tissue engineering, stem cell therapy, and genetic engineering may play a role in repairing and reviving cryopreserved individuals.

5. Artificial Intelligence (AI): AI could revolutionize cryonics by optimizing preservation protocols, predicting outcomes, and assisting in the revival process. Machine learning algorithms could analyze vast amounts of data to improve cryopreservation techniques and develop personalized revival plans.

6. Legal and Ethical Frameworks: As cryonics technology advances, there will be a need for updated legal and ethical frameworks. These frameworks will address issues such as consent, ownership of cryopreserved bodies, and the rights of revived individuals. Developing robust legal and ethical guidelines will be crucial for the responsible advancement of cryonics.

7. Public Awareness and Acceptance: Increasing public awareness and acceptance of cryonics is essential for its growth. Educational initiatives, public outreach, and transparent communication about the science and ethics of cryonics can help build trust and support for the field.

Implications for Caregivers

Advancements in cryonics technology and practice will have significant implications for social workers, doulas, caregivers, and caring others. Understanding these implications can help caregivers better support clients who choose cryonics.

1. Enhanced Knowledge and Training: Caregivers will need to stay informed about the latest developments in cryonics. Ongoing education and training will be essential to provide accurate information and effective support to clients.

2. Ethical Considerations: As cryonics technology evolves, caregivers will need to navigate new ethical considerations. This includes addressing questions about the quality of life after revival, the rights of revived individuals, and the potential societal impacts of cryonics.

3. Emotional Support: The emotional landscape of cryonics may change as technology advances. Caregivers will need to adapt their support strategies to address new hopes, fears, and uncertainties that clients and their families may experience.

4. Collaboration with Cryonics Organizations: Strong collaboration with cryonics organizations will be crucial. Caregivers should establish relationships with these organizations to ensure seamless coordination and support for clients.

5. Advocacy and Policy Development: Caregivers can play a role in advocating for ethical and legal frameworks that protect the rights and interests of cryonics clients. Involvement in policy development can help shape the future of cryonics in a responsible and ethical manner.

Conclusion

The field of cryonics is poised for significant advancements, driven by ongoing research and technological innovation. Improved cryoprotectants, nanotechnology, organ preservation, AI, and evolving legal and ethical frameworks are among the potential developments that could transform cryonics. For social workers, doulas, caregivers, and caring others, staying informed about these advancements and understanding their implications is essential. By doing so, caregivers can provide informed, compassionate, and effective support to clients exploring the possibilities of cryonics. This Section has outlined the potential future developments in cryonics technology and practice, offering a glimpse into the exciting possibilities that lie ahead.

SECTION 16: Implications for Caregivers

How these advancements might impact the roles of social workers, doulas, and caregivers.

As advancements in cryonics technology and practices continue to evolve, the roles of social workers, doulas, caregivers, and other caring professionals will inevitably be impacted. This Section explores these implications, highlighting new responsibilities, opportunities, and challenges that may arise.

Enhanced Knowledge and Training

1. Ongoing Education: Caregivers will need to stay informed about the latest developments in cryonics. This includes understanding new techniques, scientific breakthroughs, and changes in legal and ethical standards.

2. Specialized Training: Additional training programs and certifications may become necessary to equip caregivers with the skills needed to support clients considering cryonics.

Expanded Roles and Responsibilities

1. Holistic Care: As cryonics becomes more integrated into end-of-life care and end-of-life-cycle care, caregivers will need to adopt a more holistic approach, addressing both the physical and emotional needs of clients, including those young and healthy.

2. Coordination with Cryonics Providers: Caregivers will need to work closely with cryonics organizations to ensure seamless coordination of services, from initial consultations to the actual cryopreservation process.

Ethical and Legal Considerations

1. Navigating Ethical Dilemmas: Caregivers may face awkward ethical issues, such as ensuring informed consent and respecting clients' wishes regarding cryonics. They must be prepared to navigate these dilemmas with sensitivity and professionalism.

2. Legal Compliance: Understanding the legal framework surrounding cryonics in different regions will be crucial. Caregivers must ensure that all actions comply with relevant laws and regulations to protect themselves and their clients.

Emotional and Psychological Support

1. Supporting Families: Providing emotional support to families will be a key aspect of the caregiver's role. This includes helping them cope with the decision-making process, managing grief, and addressing any concerns or fears they may have.

2. Counseling Skills: Enhanced counseling skills will be essential for discussing cryonics with clients and their families, ensuring that they feel supported and informed throughout the process.

Advocacy and Public Awareness

1. Promoting Understanding: Caregivers can play a vital role in promoting public understanding of cryonics. This includes dispelling myths, providing accurate information, and advocating for the rights of individuals who choose cryonics.

2. Community Engagement: Engaging with the community through workshops, seminars, and support groups can help raise awareness and provide a platform for discussing cryonics-related issues.

Future Opportunities and Challenges

1. Technological Advancements: As cryonics technology advances, caregivers will need to adapt to new methods and practices. This may include learning about new cryopreservation techniques or understanding the implications of potential revival technologies.

2. Resource Allocation: Ensuring that adequate resources are available to support clients considering cryonics can be a challenge. This includes financial resources, access to specialized care, and support networks.

Collaboration and Networking

1. Building Networks: Establishing strong networks with other professionals in the field of cryonics will be essential. This includes collaborating with medical professionals, legal experts, and cryonics organizations to provide comprehensive support to clients.

2. Sharing Best Practices: Caregivers can benefit from sharing best practices and experiences with their peers. This can help improve the quality of care and support provided to clients considering cryonics.

Conclusion

The advancements in cryonics present both opportunities and challenges for caregivers. By staying informed, enhancing their skills, and adopting a holistic approach to care, social workers, doulas, and other caring professionals can effectively support individuals and families considering cryonics. Embracing these changes will not only improve the quality of care but also contribute to the broader acceptance and understanding of cryonics as a viable option for end-of-life planning, end-of-life-cycle preparation, and a lifestyle that is pro healthspan extension.

PART NINE: Conclusion

- **SECTION 17: Summary of Key Points**: Recap of the main points covered in the guidebook.

- **SECTION 18: Final Thoughts**: Reflections on the importance of understanding and supporting cryonics in caregiving professions.

SECTION 17: Summary of Key Points

Recap of the main points covered in the guidebook.

In this Section, we will recap the essential points covered throughout the guidebook, ensuring that social workers, doulas, caregivers, and other caring professionals have a clear understanding of cryonics and their roles in supporting individuals and families considering this option.

Purpose of the Guidebook

Need for Guidance: The guidebook addresses the growing interest in cryonics and the unique support roles that social workers, doulas, and caregivers play. It fills a gap in resources tailored to these professionals.

Overview of Cryonics

Definition and Goals: Cryonics involves preserving individuals at extremely low temperatures with the hope of future revival, aiming to extend life and cure currently incurable diseases.

History and Development

Evolution: Cryonics has evolved from early experiments in the 1960s to modern advancements, with significant milestones and contributions from key figures in the field.

Scientific Principles

Cryopreservation and Revival: The scientific basis of cryonics includes vitrification (preventing ice formation) and the theoretical potential for future revival.

Ethical Issues

Debates and Concerns: Ethical issues in cryonics include informed consent, the definition of death, and the moral implications of revival.

Legal Framework

Legal Status: The legal status of cryonics varies by region, with different regulations and implications for practitioners. One key concern is timely pronouncement of legal death and instantaneous commencement of the cryonics process.

Support and Advocacy

Role of Social Workers: Social workers can provide crucial support, advocacy, education, and emotional assistance to individuals and families considering cryonics.

Counseling Techniques

Effective Methods: Counseling techniques are essential for discussing cryonics with clients, addressing fears, misconceptions, and providing balanced information.

End-of-Life Care

Integration into Practices: Doulas can incorporate cryonics into their end-of-life care practices, ensuring a holistic approach to care that includes clients who are young and healthy. Such an approach contributes to the broader acceptance and understanding of cryonics as a viable option for end-of-life planning, end-of-life-cycle preparation, and a lifestyle that is pro healthspan extension.

Emotional Support

Supporting Families: Providing emotional support to clients and their families during the cryonics process is vital, including grief counseling and coping mechanisms.

Preparation and Planning

Steps for Cryopreservation: Detailed steps for preparing for cryopreservation, including legal, medical, and logistical arrangements, are crucial for a smooth process. (Many of these steps should be taken while the client is young and healthy.)

Communication Strategies

Best Practices: Effective communication strategies ensure clarity and empathy when discussing cryonics with clients and families.

Real-Life Examples

Case Studies: Real-life case studies highlight the experiences of individuals who have chosen cryonics and their caregivers, providing practical insights.

Lessons Learned

Insights: Key lessons from case studies offer valuable advice for practitioners, emphasizing the importance of preparation and support.

Advancements in Cryonics

Future Developments: Potential future developments in cryonics technology and practice could significantly impact the field, offering new opportunities and challenges.

Implications for Caregivers

Impact on Roles: Advancements in cryonics may affect the roles of social workers, doulas, and caregivers, introducing new responsibilities and opportunities for growth. (This could mean an increasing number of clients who are young and healthy.)

Summary of Key Points

Recap: This guidebook has provided an overview of cryonics, its scientific principles, ethical and legal considerations, and the crucial roles of social workers, doulas, and caregivers. By understanding and supporting cryonics, these professionals can better assist individuals and families in making informed decisions about their future.

This Section serves as a concise recap of the guidebook's main points, reinforcing the importance of knowledge and support in the field of cryonics.

SECTION 18: Final Thoughts

Reflections on the importance of understanding and supporting cryonics in caregiving professions.

As we approach the conclusion of this guidebook, it is important to reflect on the journey we have taken through the fascinating world of cryonics. This field, at the intersection of science, ethics, and personal choice, offers a unique perspective on life, death, and the possibilities that lie beyond our current understanding.

The Importance of Understanding Cryonics

Cryonics is more than just a scientific endeavor; it is a deeply personal choice that reflects an individual's hopes, fears, and desires for the future. For social workers, doulas, caregivers, and other caring professionals, understanding cryonics is crucial. It allows us to provide informed, compassionate support to those considering this option, ensuring that their decisions are respected and their needs are met.

Supporting Clients and Families

The role of caregivers in the cryonics process cannot be overstated. From providing emotional support to navigating ethical and legal challenges, caregivers are essential in helping clients and their families make informed decisions. By staying educated about the latest advancements and maintaining an open, empathetic approach, caregivers can offer invaluable assistance during what can be a difficult and emotional time.

Embracing Innovation and Change

Cryonics represents a frontier of medical science that encourages us to delve deeper into our notions of life and death. As this field continues to evolve, so too must our approaches to caregiving. Embracing innovation and being open to new ideas will enable us to better serve our clients and adapt to the changing landscape of end-of-life care, end-of-life-cycle care, and a lifestyle that is pro healthspan extension.

The Future of Cryonics and Caregiving

Looking ahead, the future of cryonics holds exciting possibilities. Advances in technology and science may one day make revival a reality, offering new hope to those who choose this path. For caregivers, this means staying at the forefront of these developments, continually learning and adapting to provide the best possible support.

A Commitment to Compassionate Care

At the heart of this guidebook is a commitment to compassionate care. Whether you are a social worker, doula, caregiver, or another caring professional, your role is to support and guide individuals through their cryonics journey with empathy and respect. By doing so, you honor their choices and contribute to a more understanding and supportive environment for all.

Conclusion

In conclusion, the "Cryonics Guidebook: A Resource for Social Workers, Doulas, Caregivers, and Caring Others" aims to equip you with the knowledge and tools needed to navigate the intricacies of cryonics. By understanding the scientific principles, ethical considerations, and emotional aspects of this field, you can provide comprehensive support to those considering cryonics, ensuring that their journey is as informed and compassionate as possible. Thank you for your dedication to this important work.

PART TEN: Growing a Turnkey Cryonics Network

- **SECTION 19: Resources**: List of resources for further reading and support.

- **SECTION 20: Glossary**: Definitions of key terms in cryonics.

- **SECTION 21: Information on VSED**: Cryonics and Voluntarily Stopping Eating and Drinking.

- **SECTION 22: Turnkey Cryonics**: Cryonics individualized to each unique client and circumstance is the goal of the cryonics counselor (social worker, doula, caregiver, or caring other).

APPENDIX: Example Templates for Cryonics Counselors
Sample documents and forms as suggested in Section 22.

SECTION 19: Resources

List of resources for further reading and support.

In this Section, we provide you a preliminary list of resources to further your understanding and support of cryonics. These resources include books, organizations, websites, articles, and support groups that offer valuable information and assistance for social workers, doulas, caregivers, and other caring professionals.

THE
PROSPECT
OF
IMMORTALITY

by
ROBERT C. W. ETTINGER

Plus Additional Comments By Others
"Developments In Cryonics 1964-2005"
Especially For This 21st Century Edition

Cultural Classics Series
By Ria University Press

Edited By Charles Tandy, Ph.D.

- **The Prospect of Immortality** by Robert Ettinger: A foundational 1960s text in the field of cryonics (written before the word "cryonics" had been invented) exploring the possibilities and implications of life extension through cryopreservation. (E-copy of the 1964 text available free online.) (Available for sale via online bookstores, including a translation in Traditional Chinese.)

THE PROSPECT OF IMMORTALITY
– FIFTY YEARS LATER

Edited By Charles Tandy, Ph.D.

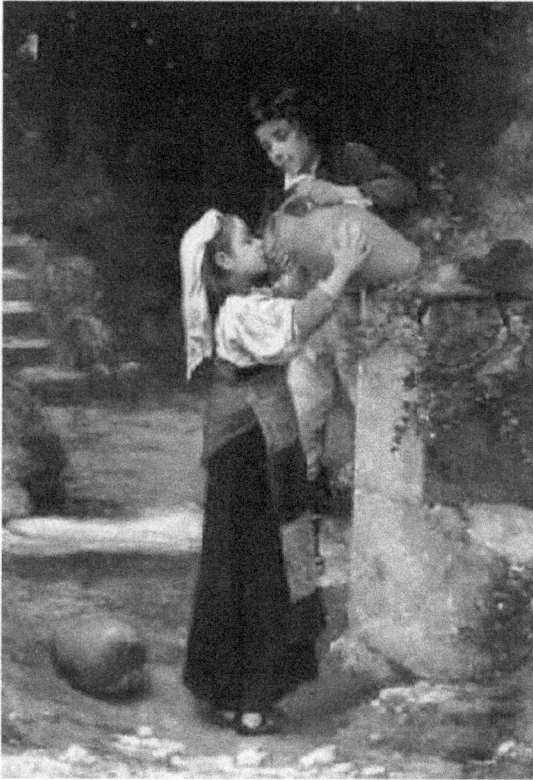

- **The Prospect of Immortality – Fifty Years Later** edited by Charles Tandy: A 500-page anthology updating Ettinger's classic work. More than a dozen contributors. (Available for sale via online bookstores.)

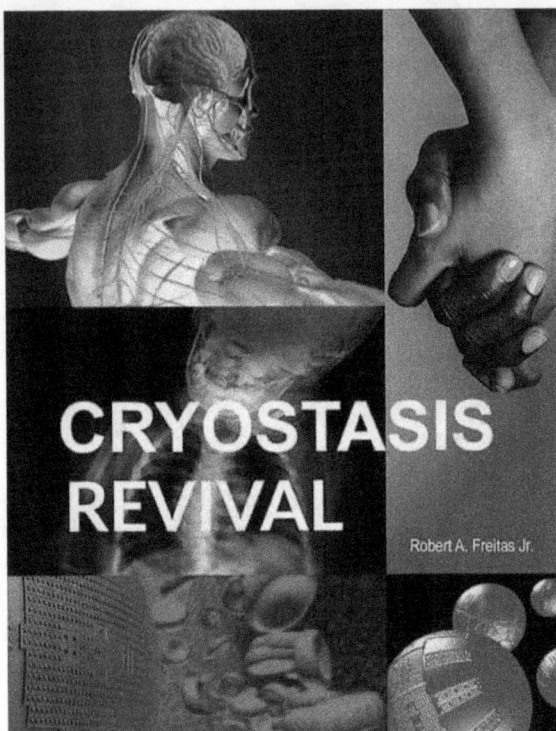

CRYOSTASIS
REVIVAL

Robert A. Freitas Jr.

- **Cryostasis Revival** by Robert A. Freitas Jr.: The processes proposed in this 700-page technical book make extensive use of a mature (future) nanotechnology and represent "the first comprehensive conceptual protocol for revival from human cryopreservation, using medical nanorobots." (E-copy available free online.) (Also available for sale via online bookstores.)

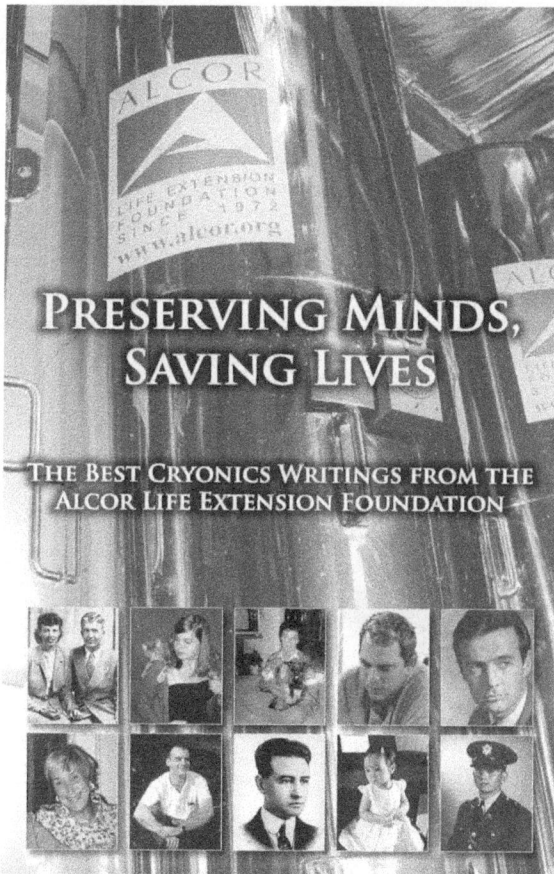

- **Preserving Minds, Saving Lives** edited by Aschwin de Wolf and Stephen Bridge: A 570-page anthology with well over a dozen contributors. From the history of the Alcor Life Extension Foundation, the editors attempt to include "the best cryonics writings." (Available for sale via online bookstores.)

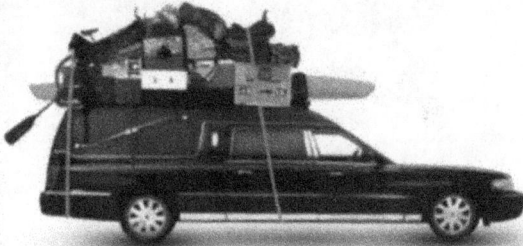

THE CRYONICS ESTATE
PLANNING HANDBOOK

MAYBE YOU CAN TAKE IT WITH YOU

RUDI HOFFMAN & PEGGY HOYT

- **The Cryonics Estate Planning Handbook: Maybe You CAN Take It with You!** by Rudi Hoffman and Peggy Hoyt: With the increasing viability of cryonics as a life-extension strategy, what if you could take your assets with you and allow the magic of compound interest to enable future revival with amazing financial options? (Available for sale via online bookstores.)

Organizations

- **Alcor Life Extension Foundation (Alcor)**: One of the leading cryonics organizations, offering cryopreservation services and conducting research into life extension technologies. (A non-profit corporation.)
- **American Cryonics Society, Inc. (ACS)**: A non-profit organization dedicated to advancing cryonics and supporting individuals who choose this option. (In the 21st century so far, less active than Alcor and CI in recruitment of new members.)
- **Cryonics Institute (CI)**: One of the leading cryonics organizations, providing cryopreservation services and promoting public awareness of cryonics. (A non-profit corporation.)
- **Others**: The present version of this Guidebook is oriented toward the United States. However, worldwide, other legitimate and active cryonics organizations exist.
- **SST Organizations**: These companies offer cryonics Standby, Stabilization, and Transportation services (costs vary).

Websites

- **Alcor.org**: The official website of the Alcor Life Extension Foundation, providing resources on cryonics, membership, and scientific research.
- **Cryonics.org**: The official website of the Cryonics Institute, offering information on their services, research, and membership options.

Journals and Articles

- **Cryobiology (Journal)**: A scientific journal that publishes research on the low temperature preservation of biological systems and on other matters related to cryobiology.

- **Cryonics Magazines**: Alcor and CI each regularly publish their own magazine for their members and the general public. (E-copies available free online.)

- **Alcor Articles and Resources**: From the Alcor Life Extension Foundation. <CryonicsArchive.org> and <Alcor.org/resources>.

- **CI Articles and Resources**: From the Cryonics Institute. <Cryonics.org/category/cryonics-library> and <Cryonics.org/all-resources>.

- **"An Open Letter to Physicians in Death-with-Dignity States (The Case of a Terminally Ill Cryonicist)"** by Charles Tandy: Available at <https://ssrn.com/abstract=2913107>.

- **"Matters Of Life And Death: Reflections On The Philosophy And Biology Of Human Cryopreservation"** by Brian Wowk: Available at <https://ssrn.com/abstract=4702055>.

- **Scientists' Open Letter on Cryonics**: Available at <https://www.biostasis.com/scientists-open-letter-on-cryonics>.

Support Groups

- **Online Forums and Discussion Groups**: Platforms such as Reddit and Facebook host various groups where individuals can discuss cryonics, share experiences, and seek advice.
- **Local Standby Groups**: These groups of volunteers, where they exist, are typically associated with Alcor and/or CI.

Educational Programs and Workshops

- **Cryonics Conferences**: Annual or periodic conferences or business meetings. Typically hosted by Alcor or the Cryonics Institute, offering opportunities for learning and networking.

- **Cryonics Workshops**: In-house training of employees (and/or volunteers) by Alcor or CI.

By utilizing these resources, social workers, doulas, caregivers, and other caring professionals can deepen their understanding of cryonics and enhance their ability to support individuals and families considering this option. Whether you are seeking scientific knowledge, ethical insights, or practical guidance, these resources can help provide a foundation for your journey into the world of cryonics.

SECTION 20: Glossary

Definitions of key terms in cryonics.

This glossary provides definitions of key terms related to cryonics, helping social workers, doulas, caregivers, and other caring professionals understand the specialized vocabulary used in this field. (Of special note below is the term "Death.")

A

• **Actual or Information Death**: Actual or Information Death (also known as Information-Theoretic Death) is not the same thing as Legal Death. Actual or Information Death is the *irreversible* loss of life, the loss of *brain structures* encoding memory and personality to the extent that it's physically impossible for *any technology* to infer them, making recovery of the original person impossible by any technology, even by the super-advanced technology of the future. (Also see "Death.")
• **Alcor Life Extension Foundation (Alcor)**: One of the leading cryonics organizations, offering cryopreservation services and conducting research into life extension technologies. (A non-profit corporation.)
• **American Cryonics Society, Inc. (ACS)**: A non-profit organization dedicated to advancing cryonics and supporting individuals who choose this option. (In the 21st century so far, less active than Alcor and CI in recruitment of new members.)

B

• **Biostasis**: The state in which biological processes are halted or greatly slowed, often used in the context of cryopreservation (cryostasis) to describe the condition of preserved tissues or organisms. (Also see "Cryonic Preservation.")

- **Brain Death**: In the mid 20th century it was observed that sometimes the brain would begin decomposing even if the heart and rest of the body remained functioning. This became called "brain death." (Also see "Cryonics and the Two Modes of Legal Death.")

C

- **Cardiopulmonary Death**: See "Clinical or Cardiopulmonary Death."
- **Caregivers**: Persons who tend to the needs or concerns of those with short- or long-term limitations, such as illness, injury or disability, including those with end-of-life-cycle needs or concerns related to cryonics.
- **Clinical Death**: See "Clinical or Cardiopulmonary Death."
- **Clinical or Cardiopulmonary Death**: Clinical or Cardiopulmonary Death is determined by cessation of breathing and heartbeat according to presently existing law including what resuscitation measures are *available or intended, if any*. (Also see "Cryonics and the Two Modes of Legal Death.")
- **Cryobiology**: The study of the effects of low temperatures on biological systems such as living organisms, tissues, and cells.
- **Cryogenics**: A branch of physics that deals with the production and effects of very low temperatures (not to be confused with either cryobiology or cryonics).
- **Cryonic Hibernation**: See "Cryonic Preservation."
- **Cryonic Preservation**: Experimental preservation of individuals at extremely low temperatures with the hope of future revival to full health (to wellness or even to better-than-wellness). The distinction in cryonics between (actual) death and legal death suggests thinking in terms of putting life on hold, the pausing of life. Thus some cryonicists will use terms like cryonic hibernation, cryonic suspension, and so on.
- **Cryonic Suspension**: See "Cryonic Preservation."
- **Cryonics**: The experimental practice of preserving individuals at extremely low temperatures with the hope of future revival. If the *cryonics patient* is legally dead, then there is an

established cryonics protocol to treat the patient as a sick person rather than as a dead corpse – for example, cryobiological vitrification (ice-free cryopreservation). Long term cryonics care means no further deterioration. *Future developments may allow inference to healthy brain structure, and recovery of the original person to full health.*

• **Cryonics and the Two Modes of Legal Death**: (1) Brain Death is a disaster for cryonics. *Cryonics patients are not to be maintained on a ventilator or other life support if their prognosis for brain recovery is poor.* (2) Clinical or Cardiopulmonary Death is NOT NECESSARILY a disaster for cryonics. A brain injured by many minutes of stopped blood circulation is a very sick brain; only much later does it become a dead brain.

• **Cryonics Institute (CI)**: One of the leading cryonics organizations, providing cryopreservation services and promoting public awareness of cryonics. (A non-profit corporation.)

• **Cryopreservation**: The process of cooling and preserving (maintaining) biological systems (such as cells, tissues, organs, or organisms) at very low temperatures to sustain their viability.

• **Cryoprotectant**: A substance used to protect biological systems from freezing damage during cryopreservation.

• **Cryostasis**: See "Biostasis."

D

• **Death**: The distinction between *legal death* and *actual death* is crucial in cryonics. Legal death is a determination of death for legal purposes. Death (actual death) is the irreversible loss of life. (Many meanings given to death, such as when used with a variety of adjectives, are not consistent with the meaning of actual death.) Death is the (absolutely) irreversible loss of life, making recovery of the original person impossible by any technology, even by the super-technology of the future. Many cryonicists today would define (actual) death as the loss of brain structures encoding memory and personality to an extent that it's physically impossible for any technology, no matter how super-advanced, to infer them. The distinction in cryonics between death and legal death suggests thinking in terms of putting life on hold, the pausing of life. Thus some cryonicists will use terms like cryonic hibernation, cryonic suspension, and so on.

- **Doulas**: There are different types of doulas. It is specifically an end-of-life-cycle doula who can assist the cryonics client. A doula is not a medical professional, but a health professional, and may work with a medical or palliative or hospice team. An end-of-life-cycle doula might work with a person or family for weeks, months, or even years. Support might include Advocacy, Companionship, Spiritual support, Grief support, Physical care, Creating a soothing environment, Cryonics planning, and more.

E

- **Ethical Issues**: In cryonics, moral inquiry and discourse surrounding the practice of cryonics, including informed consent, the definition of death, and the implications of future revival.

F

- **Freezing Damage**: Damage caused to biological systems by the formation of ice crystals during the cooling process. In cryonics, cryoprotectants are used to minimize this damage.

H

- **Hypothermia**: A medical condition in which the body temperature drops below the normal range, often used in cryonics to describe the initial cooling process before cryopreservation.

I

- **Immortality**: In **The Prospect of Immortality** by Robert Ettinger, immortality means indefinitely long and healthy life.
- **Information Death** or **Information-Theoretic Death**: See "Actual or Information Death."
- **Informed Consent**: The process of obtaining voluntary agreement (from a sufficiently competent person) after they have

been informed of all the potential risks and benefits of a procedure or treatment.

L

- **Legal Death**: Legal Death is NOT the same thing as Actual or Information Death. Legal Death is a determination of death for *legal* purposes. In the United States there are two methods by which legal death can be pronounced: (1) Brain Death; and, (2) Clinical or Cardiopulmonary Death. Also see "Death."
- **Legal Framework**: In cryonics, the set of laws and regulations governing the practice of cryonics in different regions. (For example, different hospitals or hospices may have differing customs, habits, procedures, rules, or regulations.)
- **Life on Hold:** Cryonics attempts to pause life for future revival to youthful health.
- **Local Standby Groups**: These groups of volunteers, where they exist, are typically associated with Alcor and/or CI. They seek to provide support and aid (bedside standby and/or stabilization and/or transportation assistance) to those locally in need of emergency cryonics services until (say) Alcor or CI can provide their professional expertise. Surrounding the time of legal death, standby and stabilization are needed if the patient is to undergo a smooth, quality cryonics process. (If one pays for standby service, this can be costly. Hence, the potential importance of local volunteers. Also, it is important to be treated as a patient, not as a corpse. One may want to form one's own local standby group or mutual aid society.)

M

- **Molecular Repair**: The theoretical process of repairing biological systems at the molecular level, which may be necessary for the revival of cryopreserved individuals.

P

- **Preservation**: In biology, the act of maintaining the condition of biological systems, such as through the use of low temperatures.

R

- **Revival**: In cryonics, the theoretical process of restoring a cryopreserved individual to healthy life (such as in a decade or a century or a millennium).
- **Rewarming**: In cryobiology, the process of raising the temperature of cryopreserved systems, such as to restore them to a functional state.

S

- **Social Workers**: Social workers are mental health professionals who work with individuals and communities to overcome challenges and effect social change. They seek to understand human problems (such as by utilizing social theories) to help improve people's lives, and to improve society as a whole. They provide support and advocacy for individuals and families, including those considering cryonics.
- **Support Groups**: Cryonics support groups provide emotional and informational support to individuals and families considering cryonics.

T

- **Transhumanism**: A philosophical movement that advocates for the use of technology to enhance human physical and cognitive abilities, often associated with the goals of cryonics or with a pro healthspan extension lifestyle.

V

- **Vitrification**: A method of cryopreservation that prevents ice formation by turning biological systems into a glass-like state.
- **Voluntarily Stopping Eating and Drinking (VSED)**: A legal and ethical end-of-life option where a person chooses to hasten death by refusing food and fluids. This can intersect with cryonics as part of an individual's end-of-life-cycle plan and pro healthspan extension lifestyle. "SED by AD" may be preferable to "VSED" if one utilizes an Advance Directive as part of one's pro healthspan extension lifestyle.

By familiarizing yourself with the terms above, you will be better equipped to understand and discuss cryonics with clients, colleagues, and other professionals. This glossary serves as a handy reference to clarify the language sometimes used in the field of cryonics.

SECTION 21: Information on VSED

Cryonics and Voluntarily Stopping Eating and Drinking.

Voluntarily Stopping Eating and Drinking (VSED) is an end-of-life option that some individuals choose to hasten death in a legal and ethical manner. This Section explores the intersection of VSED and cryonics as part of an individual's end-of-life-cycle plan and pro healthspan extension lifestyle, providing caregivers with the information needed to support clients who may consider both options. **Incorporating VSED/SED into one's Cryonics Advance Directive while one is young and healthy is found desirable by some practitioners of healthspan extension.**

Understanding VSED

- **Definition**: VSED involves a conscious decision, such as by a terminally ill or severely suffering (but sufficiently competent) individual, to stop eating and drinking, leading to legal death from dehydration. It is legal in all 50 states of the United States and may be considered a form of palliative care.

- **Process**: The process typically involves the individual making an informed decision, often with the support of healthcare professionals, family members, and caregivers. The individual stops all intake of food and fluids, and death (in its legal meaning) usually occurs within one to three weeks.

Cryonics and VSED

- **Compatibility**: While VSED and cryonics may seem contradictory, they can be part of a comprehensive end-of-life-cycle plan. An individual may choose VSED to control the timing of their legal death, followed instantaneously by the cryonics process to preserve their body for potential future revival to health.
- **Planning**: Integrating VSED with cryonics requires careful planning. This includes ensuring that the commencement of the cryonics process begins instantaneously upon immediate official declaration of legal death.

Support for VSED and Cryonics

- **Role of Caregivers**: Caregivers play a crucial role in supporting individuals who choose VSED and cryonics. This includes providing emotional support, ensuring comfort, and coordinating with medical and cryonics professionals.
- **Emotional Support**: Supporting clients and their families through the VSED-cryonics process involves addressing fears, providing reassurance, and helping them cope with the emotional aspects of the decision.

Ethical and Legal Considerations

- **Informed Consent**: Ensuring that the individual has made an informed decision is paramount. This involves discussing the implications of VSED and cryonics, including the potential outcomes and ethical considerations.
- **Legal Compliance**: Caregivers must be aware of the legal status of VSED and cryonics in their region. This includes understanding the requirements for **immediate** declaration of **legal**

death, the documenting of informed consent, and the coordinating of healthcare providers and cryonics organizations.

Case Studies

- **Real-Life Examples**: Examining case studies of individuals who have chosen VSED and cryonics can provide valuable insights. These examples highlight the practical challenges and successes of integrating these end-of-life-cycle options.
- **Lessons Learned**: Without doubt, key lessons from these case studies include the importance of clear communication, thorough planning, and compassionate support.

Practical Guidance

- **Communication Strategies**: Effective communication is essential when discussing VSED and cryonics with clients and their families. This includes being honest, empathetic, and providing clear information about the dual process and its implications.
- **Coordination with Professionals**: Working closely with medical professionals, legal advisors, and cryonics organizations ensures that the individual's wishes are respected and that the process is carried out smoothly as part of an individual's end-of-life-cycle plan and pro healthspan extension lifestyle.

Conclusion

VSED and cryonics represent two distinct yet potentially complementary options. By understanding the nuances of both, caregivers can provide comprehensive support to individuals and families considering these choices. This Section aims to equip caregivers with the knowledge and tools needed to begin navigating the duel VSED-cryonics process, ensuring that their clients' decisions are respected and their needs are met with compassion and professionalism.

SECTION 22: Turnkey Cryonics

Cryonics individualized to each unique client and circumstance is the goal of the cryonics counselor (social worker, doula, caregiver, or caring other).

Introduction

The goal of a turnkey cryonics network is to provide a seamless, comprehensive service that addresses the unique needs and circumstances of each client. This Section will explore the steps necessary to establish and grow such a network, emphasizing the importance of individualized care and the critical role of cryonics counselors, including social workers, doulas, caregivers, and other caring professionals. Not to be overlooked is that many cryonics clients are young and healthy. Also not to be overlooked is that there are about as many animals (pets) in cryonic preservation as humans.

Understanding Turnkey Cryonics

Turnkey cryonics refers to a fully integrated service that manages all aspects of the cryonics process, from initial consultation to standby to cryopreservation to long-term cryonics care. This approach ensures that clients receive personalized support tailored to their specific needs, preferences, and circumstances.

Key Components of a Turnkey Cryonics Network

1.   **Comprehensive Assessment**: Conduct thorough assessments to understand each client's medical history, personal preferences, and end-of-life-cycle wishes. This information is crucial for creating a personalized cryonics plan.
2.   **Education and Counseling**: Provide clients and their families with detailed information about cryonics, including the scientific principles, potential benefits, and ethical considerations. Counseling services should address any emotional or psychological concerns.

3.   **Legal and Ethical Considerations**: Ensure that all legal documents, such as consent forms and advance directives, are in place. Address ethical issues related to cryonics, including informed consent and the rights of the client.

4.   **Medical and Technical Support**: Collaborate with medical professionals to manage the client's health and prepare for the cryonics process. This includes coordinating with cryonics facilities and ensuring that all technical aspects are handled efficiently.

5.   **Emotional and Psychological Support**: Offer ongoing emotional and psychological support to clients and their families. This can include grief counseling, support groups, and other resources to help them cope with the process.

6.   **Logistics and Coordination**: Manage all logistical aspects of the cryonics process, including bedside standby, stabilization, transportation, cryopreservation, and long term cryonics care of the client/patient. Ensure that all procedures are carried out smoothly and efficiently.

The Role of Cryonics Counselors

Cryonics counselors, including social workers, doulas, caregivers, and other caring professionals, play a pivotal role in the turnkey cryonics network. Their responsibilities include:

1.   **Client Advocacy**: Act as advocates for clients, ensuring their wishes and needs are respected throughout the cryonics process. This includes facilitating communication between clients, families, and medical professionals.

2.   **Personalized Care Plans**: Develop and implement individualized care plans that address the unique circumstances of each client. This involves coordinating with various stakeholders to ensure all aspects of the client's care are covered.

3.   **Emotional Support**: Provide emotional and psychological support to clients and their families. Cryonics counselors help clients navigate the emotional challenges of the cryonics process, offering empathy and understanding.

4.   **Education and Outreach**: Educate clients, families, and the broader community about cryonics. This includes dispelling

myths, providing accurate information, and raising awareness about the benefits and challenges of cryonics.

5.	**Coordination and Logistics**: Oversee the logistical aspects of the cryonics process, ensuring that all procedures are carried out efficiently and in accordance with the client's wishes. This includes coordinating of bedside standby, stabilization, transportation, cryopreservation, and long term cryonics care of the client/patient.

6.	**Continuous Support**: Offer ongoing support to clients and their families. Ensure that clients and their loved ones feel supported throughout the entire process. (This may include post-cryopreservation care and follow-up.)

Individualized Cryonics Plans

Creating individualized cryonics plans is essential to meet the unique needs and preferences of each client. These plans should be comprehensive and adaptable, covering all aspects of the cryonics process. Key elements include:

1.	**Personal Preferences**: Document the client's specific wishes regarding their cryonics process, including any personal, cultural, or spiritual considerations.

2.	**Medical History**: Include relevant medical history to inform the cryonics team of any conditions or treatments that may affect the cryonics process.

3.	**Legal Documentation**: Ensure all necessary legal documents are completed and accessible, including consent forms and advance directives.

4.	**Emergency Procedures**: Outline clear instructions for emergency situations, including contact information for key individuals and organizations.

5.	**Post-Cryopreservation Plans**: Detail any specific wishes for post-cryopreservation care and follow-up, ensuring that the client's preferences are respected.

Building a Network

1.   **Partnerships and Collaborations**: Establish partnerships with medical professionals, cryonics facilities, legal experts, and other relevant organizations. Collaboration is key to providing comprehensive care and building a turnkey cryonics network.
2.   **Training and Certification**: Develop training programs for cryonics counselors to ensure they have the necessary skills and knowledge. Certification can help maintain high standards of cryonics care.
3.   **Community Outreach and Education**: Raise awareness about cryonics through community outreach and education programs. This can help build trust and attract potential clients.
4.   **Continuous Improvement**: Regularly evaluate and improve the services offered by the network. Gather feedback from clients and their families to identify areas for improvement.

Case Studies and Examples

Include case studies and examples of successful turnkey cryonics projects and networks. Highlight best practices and lessons learned to provide practical insights for building and growing a network.

Conclusion

Growing a turnkey cryonics network requires a holistic approach that addresses the unique needs of each client. Not to be overlooked is that many cryonics clients are young and healthy. Also not to be overlooked is that there are about as many animals (family pets) in cryonic preservation as humans. By focusing on individualized care, collaboration, and continuous improvement, cryonics counselors can provide a valuable service that supports clients and their families through the cryonics process.

APPENDIX: Example Templates for Cryonics Counselors

Sample documents and forms as suggested in Section 22.

Below, you'll find templates and examples of essential documents and forms that cryonics counselors can use to streamline their processes and ensure comprehensive care for their clients. Not to be overlooked is that many cryonics clients are young and healthy. Also not to be overlooked is that there are about as many animals (family pets) in cryonic preservation as humans. To facilitate the creation and management of individualized cryonics plans, the following sample documents and forms are provided. These samples can be customized to fit the specific needs and circumstances of each client.

Client Intake Form

Personal Information

Name

Date of Birth

Address

Phone Number

Email

Medical History

Primary Physician

Current Medications

Known Allergies

Medical Conditions

Emergency Contacts

Name

Relationship

Phone Number

Email

Cryonics Preferences

Preferred Cryonics Facility

Specific Instructions

Additional Notes

Cryonics Plan Agreement

This agreement outlines the terms and conditions of the cryonics plan between the client and the cryonics provider.

Parties Involved:

Client Name:

Cryonics Provider:

Terms and Conditions:

1. **Services Provided**: The cryonics provider agrees to perform cryopreservation services as outlined in the client's individualized cryonics plan.

2. **Payment**: The client agrees to pay the specified fees for cryopreservation services.

3. **Legal Compliance**: Both parties agree to comply with all relevant legal and regulatory requirements.

Signatures:

Client Signature:
Date:

Cryonics Provider Signature:
Date:

Emergency Contact and Standby Instructions

In the event of an emergency, please contact those listed below and follow these instructions:

Primary Contact:

Name:

Relationship:

Phone Number:

Email:

Secondary Contact:

Name:

Relationship:

Phone Number:

Email:

Standby Instructions:

1. **Initial Notification**: Contact the primary emergency contact immediately.
2. **Cryonics Facility Notification**: Notify the designated cryonics facility of the client's condition.
3. **Medical Personnel Coordination**: Coordinate with medical personnel to ensure proper handling and preparation for cryopreservation.
4. **Transportation Arrangements**: Arrange for transportation to the cryonics facility per the client's cryonics plan.

Legal and Financial Checklist

Ensure the following documents are completed and accessible:

1. **Legal Documents:**
   Consent Forms
   Advance Directives
   Power of Attorney
   Will

2. **Financial Documents:**
   Payment Arrangements
   Insurance Policies
   Trusts and Estates

3. **Cryonics Plan Documents:**
   Cryonics Plan Agreement
   Emergency Contact and Standby Instructions
   Post-Cryopreservation Follow-Up Form

4. **Additional Considerations:**
   □ **Ensure** all documents are properly witnessed and/or notarized (as required or desirable).
   □ **Keep** copies of all documents in a secure and accessible location.
   □ **Inform** relevant parties (family, legal representatives) of the location of these documents.
   □ **Consider** storing documents, such as the advance directive, with the U.S. Advance Care Plan Registry® ($49.95, lifetime registration) at <https://www.usacpr.com>.
   □ **Consider** filing a "Human Cryopreservation Response Team Application" to help in local cryonics emergencies (non-medical folks should check the VOLUNTEER box): CryoRegistry <https://www.biostasistechnologies.org/registry>.

Post-Cryopreservation Follow-Up Form

This form documents the client's wishes for post-cryopreservation care and follow-up.

Client Information

Name

Date of Birth

Cryonics Facility

Post-Cryopreservation Instructions

Preferred Contact for Updates

Frequency of Updates

Specific Instructions for Care

Additional Notes

Signatures

Client Signature

Date

Cryonics Provider Signature

Date

Cryonics Advance Directive for Health Care
(State of Michigan Template)

The cryonics template below is based on my (Charles Tandy's) own legal document. I thank Brian Wowk for his assistance – see his paper at (https://ssrn.com/abstract=4702055).

Please use this (Advance Directive for Health Care) template as you wish. The document complies with all Michigan state legal requirements. It may of course be wise to reformat the document to fit your own font style, paper size, etc. This example lists four patient advocates, but the number of patient advocates is up to the client (so long as there is at least one patient advocate). **If you are not a Michigander, your legal requirements may differ.**

Durable Power of Attorney for Health Care (DPOA-HC)
State of Michigan
Advance Directive and Patient Advocate
Life-Sustaining Treatment and Scope of Treatment
Patient: Charles E. Tandy (DOB: **/**/****)

Part A: Make Your Health Care Wishes Known

Honoring someone's "last wishes" is seen as a benevolent duty in America and many other cultures. I ask that my "last wishes" be honored with an emphasis on the protocol described below.

CONCERNS:

> Standard formats may not adequately address the circumstances of the cryonics patient. *A critical task in cryonics advance planning is to clarify the patient's values, goals and wishes that the patient wants others to follow.*

> Hopefully this document will also help correct misinformation about cryonics.

- 100 -

> Please note that the biomedical technical papers about cryonics in the PubMed literature speak favorably of its eventual success (https://ssrn.com/abstract=2913107). Also worth noting is the Scientists' Open Letter on Cryonics (https://cryonics.org/cryonics-library/scientists-open-letter-on-cryonics).

TERMINOLOGIES:

> **Actual or Information Death** is not the same thing as Legal Death. **Actual or Information Death** is the *irreversible* loss of life. **Actual or Information Death** is the loss of *brain structures* encoding memory and personality to the extent that it's physically impossible for *any technology* to infer them, making recovery of the original person impossible by any technology, even the super-advanced technology of the future.

> **Legal Death** is NOT the same thing as Actual or Information Death. **Legal Death** is a determination of death for *legal* purposes. In the United States, there are two methods by which legal death can be pronounced: (1) **Brain Death**; and, (2) **Clinical or Cardiopulmonary Death**.

> **Brain Death**: In the mid-20th century it was observed that sometimes the brain would begin decomposing even if the heart and rest of the body remained functioning. This became called "brain death."

> **Clinical or Cardiopulmonary Death** is determined by cessation of breathing and heartbeat according to presently existing law including what resuscitation measures are *available or intended, if any*.

> **Cryonics**: If the *cryonics patient* is legally dead, then there is an established cryonics protocol to treat the patient as a sick person rather than as a corpse – for example, cryobiological vitrification (ice-free cryopreservation). Long-term cryonics care means no further deterioration. *Future developments may allow inference to healthy brain structure, and recovery of the original person to full health.*

- 101 -

> **Cryonics and the Two Modes of Legal Death**: (1) **Brain Death** is a disaster for cryonics. *Cryonics patients are not to be maintained on a ventilator or other life support if their prognosis for brain recovery is poor.* (2) **Clinical or Cardiopulmonary Death** is NOT NECESSARILY a disaster for cryonics. A brain injured by many minutes of stopped blood circulation is a very sick brain; only much later does it become a dead brain.

The Patient (Charles E. Tandy) hereby directs everyone -- specifically including physicians, nurses, and other health care providers – to honor the concerns and terminologies mentioned above.

Ideally, the cryonics patient will at NO point undergo FREEZING – but will, instead, initially undergo cooling to 34°F (1°C) and later undergo cryobiological vitrification (ice-free cryopreservation rather than freezing).

Ideally, the legal death of the patient (Charles E. Tandy) is followed INSTANTANEOUSLY by cryonics measures **that treat the patient as a person (as an ONGOING patient, not as a corpse).** If the cryonics patient is legally dead, then there is an established cryonics protocol to treat the patient as a person rather than as a corpse. This eventually involves cooling of the patient to cryogenic temperature such as via cryobiological vitrification (ice-free cryopreservation). Then the patient is placed in long-term cryonics care at cryogenic temperature (such as via liquid nitrogen). This means no further deterioration, thus the patient is waiting for future technological, medical, and rejuvenation developments. Such future developments may allow inference to healthy brain structure, and recovery of the original person to full health.

Whole Body Donor – URGENT!

Do NOT Autopsy! Do NOT Embalm! Do NOT Freeze!

In the event of CRITICAL ILLNESS, clinical death, legal death, or cardiopulmonary death, please call the numbers listed below until someone answers:
Cryonics Institute (CI).....586 791-5961
CI Toll-Free.....866 288-2796
CI Emergency.....586 817-0926

In the event of clinical/legal/cardiopulmonary death:
<u>**Immediately cool the patient (e.g. with bags of crushed ice),**</u>
<u>**especially the head,**</u>
<u>**and follow the Cryonics Institute instructions.**</u>

Do NOT Autopsy! Do NOT Embalm! Do NOT Freeze!
Uniform Anatomical Gift Act
Whole Body Donor To
Cryonics Institute (Clinton Township, Michigan) Cryonics.org

If I'm neurologically injured or otherwise neurologically compromised with a poor prognosis, then I request comfort care only and withdrawal of all life support including food and fluids. Life support may be continued for a limited time at the request of the Cryonics Institute for the sole purpose of facilitating the logistics of my cryopreservation by **controlling the timing of my legal death.**

It's my strong wish that legal death be pronounced as soon as possible after cessation of heartbeat determined by auscultation so that cooling and other procedures to facilitate my cryopreservation can begin as soon as possible. **Under NO circumstances should I be allowed to become legally brain dead** (e.g., while on life support); see above.

Please work with the Cryonics Institute to optimize the timing of my legal death.

I ask for the fullest possible cooperation with the Cryonics Institute with whom I have legal arrangements for cryopreservation, with the personnel they may send to facilitate that process, and with the provision of my personal medical information as requested by that organization and its personnel before and after my legal death, which I hereby authorize.

The cryonics patient (Charles E. Tandy) wants physicians, nurses, health care providers – and everyone else – to follow the patient's values, goals, and wishes expressed in the present document.

PERSONAL EMERGENCY CONTACTS FOR CHARLES E. TANDY

(1) Name: Andy Zawacki
Relationship: Friend
Address: Cryonics Institute: 24355 Sorrentino Court, Clinton
          Township, Michigan 48035-3239
Telephone: 586 791-5961; 866 288-2796; 586 817-0926
Email: info@cryonics.org
Website: Cryonics.org

(2) Name: ******
Relationship: ******
Address: ******
          ******
Telephone: ******
Email: ******
Website: ******

Additional Instructions: Procedures for Medical Facilities (Hospitals, Hospices, Etc.)

"DONORS AFTER CARDIAC DEATH ARE NOT DEAD." This is an all-caps section heading in a mainstream medical journal article discussing cardiopulmonary death in the context of organ donation (https://ssrn.com/abstract=4702055). Concerning *long-term* whole-organ cryopreservation for transplantation, Dr. Michael J. Taylor (Chief Science Officer at Sylvatica Biotech, Inc.) has pointed out: "Progress in developing appropriate cooling technologies to achieve vitrification [ice-free cryopreservation] has advanced more rapidly than complimentary warming techniques, which now present the principle stumbling block."

The brain is a very special organ – please note the special importance of the timing of my legal death so that cooling and cryonics measures begin INSTANTANEOUSLY, treating me as an ONGOING patient, not as a corpse.

Please work with the Cryonics Institute to optimize the TIMING of my legal death.

Please work with the Cryonics Institute to optimize my ONGOING medical care.

Upon clinical death, the following should be done IMMEDIATELY:

1.   Cool patient by TOPICAL APPLICATION OF ICE or other coolant, WITH SPECIAL ATTENTION TO THE HEAD -- e.g., bags of crushed ice.

2.   Please LEAVE IN PLACE ANY ACCESS OR DRAINAGE TUBES, such as I.V., N.G., Foley, and/or tracheotomy tube with oxygen line. If an I.V. line is not in place, please insert one.

3.   ADMINISTER HEPARIN (INTRAVENOUSLY IF POSSIBLE). Use 30,000 units (40,000 units if the patient is over 200 pounds).

4.   If possible, after the pronouncement of legal death, use prompt CPR-like compressions to MAINTAIN HEART AND LUNG FUNCTION. Vigorous compressions for 5 to 15 minutes are to delay deterioration, improve heat transfer, and circulate heparin throughout the body. (Yes, "vigorous" is best even if it means breaking ribs.)

5.   CALL CRYONICS INSTITUTE EMERGENCY TELEPHONE NUMBERS BELOW UNTIL CRYONICS INSTITUTE PERSONNEL ARE ALERTED:

- **Cryonics Institute: 586 791-5961**
- **Facility Manager: 586 817-0926**

RELEASE PATIENT WITH NO DELAY TO CRYONICS INSTITUTE PERSONNEL upon their arrival. *Your help is sincerely appreciated!*

Instructions to Patient Advocate

I want my Patient Advocate to make decisions about life-sustaining treatment and scope of treatment. When making these decisions, I want my Patient Advocate to follow the guidelines I have provided.

{_____}
Signature of Charles E. Tandy

Part B: Appoint a Patient Advocate

Patient: Charles E. Tandy (DOB: **/**/****)

(1) I want this person to be my Patient Advocate if I can no longer make my medical decisions for myself:
Name: ******
Address: ******
Telephone: ******

(2) If the above person cannot do it, then I want the following person to make my medical decisions when I cannot and be my successor Patient Advocate:
Name: ******
Address: ******
Telephone: ******

(3) If the above person cannot do it, then I want the following person to make my medical decisions when I cannot and be my successor Patient Advocate:
Name: ******
Address: ******
Telephone: ******

(4) If the above person cannot do it, then I want the following person to make my medical decisions when I cannot and be my successor Patient Advocate:
Name: ******
Address: ******
Telephone: ******

Part C: Signatures

Signature of Charles E. Tandy:

{_____}

  Signature   Date

(Name and Address:)
Charles E. Tandy
******
******
(Date of Birth:)
//****

Witnesses' Signatures:

By signing, I promise that Charles E. Tandy signed this form while I watched; Charles E. Tandy appeared to be thinking clearly and was not forced to sign.

Witness #1

{_____}

  Sign Your Name   Date

{_____}

  Print Your First Name   Print Your Last Name

{_____}

  Street Address   City   State   Zip

Witness #2

{_____}
  Sign Your Name   Date

{_____}
  Print Your First Name   Print Your Last Name

{_____}
  Street Address   City   State   Zip

Part D: Acceptance by Patient Advocate (Durable Power of Attorney for Health Care)

As the Patient Advocate (Surrogate Decision Maker)

Based on the wishes of Charles E. Tandy, you can *agree to, say no to, change, stop, or choose:*

- Doctors, nurses, social workers, health care providers; Hospitals, clinics, nursing homes, hospices, abodes; Medications, tests, treatments; Life support related issues; Surgery related issues; Comfort care and hospice care issues. *You may look at the medical records of Charles E. Tandy to help you make these decisions on behalf of the patient.*

Specific instructions regarding Life-Sustaining Treatment and Scope of Treatment:

- You will follow the guidelines that the patient (Charles E. Tandy) has provided.

Generic instructions as the Patient Advocate:

- You should always act with the patient's best interests and not your own interests.

- You will only start making decisions for the patient after 2 doctors agree that the patient is too sick to make his or her own decisions.

- You will not be able to make decisions that the patient would not usually be able to make.

- You don't have the power to stop a pregnant patient's treatment if it would cause her to die.

- You can make a decision to stop or not start treatments and allow the patient to die naturally if they have made it clear that you can make that decision.

- You cannot be paid for your role as a Patient Advocate but you can get paid back for the money you spend on the patient's medical expenses.

- You should help to protect the patient's rights as defined by law.

- You cannot make decisions that go against the patients' wishes regarding organ donation.

- The patient can remove you as Patient Advocate whenever they want.

- You can remove yourself as Patient Advocate whenever you want.

By signing, I am saying that I understand what this document says and that I will be the Patient Advocate for Charles E. Tandy.

Durable Power of Attorney for Health Care (DPOA-HC)
Patient Advocate (Surrogate Decision Maker) List

Patient Advocate: ****
Address: ******
Telephone: ******

2nd Patient Advocate: ****
Address: ******
Telephone: ******

3rd Patient Advocate: ****
Address: ******
Telephone: ******

4th Patient Advocate: ****
Address: ******
Telephone: ******

Signatures: See the following pages.

As the Patient Advocate (Surrogate Decision Maker)

Based on the wishes of Charles E. Tandy, you can *agree to, say no to, change, stop, or choose:*

- Doctors, nurses, social workers, health care providers; Hospitals, clinics, nursing homes, hospices, abodes; Medications, tests, treatments; Life support related issues; Surgery related issues; Comfort care and hospice care issues. *You may look at the medical records of Charles E. Tandy to help you make these decisions on behalf of the patient.*

Specific instructions regarding Life-Sustaining Treatment and Scope of Treatment:

- You will follow the guidelines that the patient (Charles E. Tandy) has provided.

Generic instructions as the Patient Advocate:

- You should always act with the patient's best interests and not your own interests.

- You will only start making decisions for the patient after 2 doctors agree that the patient is too sick to make his or her own decisions.

- You will not be able to make decisions that the patient would not usually be able to make.

- You don't have the power to stop a pregnant patient's treatment if it would cause her to die.

- You can make a decision to stop or not start treatments and allow the patient to die naturally if they have made it clear that you can make that decision.

- You cannot be paid for your role as a Patient Advocate but you can get paid back for the money you spend on the patient's medical expenses.

- You should help to protect the patient's rights as defined by law.

- You cannot make decisions that go against the patients' wishes regarding organ donation.

- The patient can remove you as Patient Advocate whenever they want.

- You can remove yourself as Patient Advocate whenever you want.

By signing, I am saying that I understand what this document says and that I will be the Patient Advocate for Charles E. Tandy.

{Patient Advocate's Signature: Date: }
Name: ******
Address: ******
Telephone: ******

As the Patient Advocate (Surrogate Decision Maker)
– 2nd Patient Advocate: ****** –

Based on the wishes of Charles E. Tandy, you can *agree to, say no to, change, stop, or choose:*

- Doctors, nurses, social workers, health care providers; Hospitals, clinics, nursing homes, hospices, abodes; Medications, tests, treatments; Life support related issues; Surgery related issues; Comfort care and hospice care issues. *You may look at the medical records of Charles E. Tandy to help you make these decisions on behalf of the patient.*

Specific instructions regarding Life-Sustaining Treatment and Scope of Treatment:

- You will follow the guidelines that the patient (Charles E. Tandy) has provided.

Generic instructions as the Patient Advocate:

- You should always act with the patient's best interests and not your own interests.

- You will only start making decisions for the patient after 2 doctors agree that the patient is too sick to make his or her own decisions.

- You will not be able to make decisions that the patient would not usually be able to make.

- You don't have the power to stop a pregnant patient's treatment if it would cause her to die.

- You can make a decision to stop or not start treatments and allow the patient to die naturally if they have made it clear that you can make that decision.

- You cannot be paid for your role as a Patient Advocate but you can get paid back for the money you spend on the patient's medical expenses.

- You should help to protect the patient's rights as defined by law.

- You cannot make decisions that go against the patients' wishes regarding organ donation.

- The patient can remove you as Patient Advocate whenever they want.

- You can remove yourself as Patient Advocate whenever you want.

By signing, I am saying that I understand what this document says and that I will be the Patient Advocate for Charles E. Tandy.

{2nd Patient Advocate's Signature: _____ Date: _____ }

Name: ******
Address: ******
Telephone: ******

As the Patient Advocate (Surrogate Decision Maker)
– 3rd Patient Advocate: ****** –

Based on the wishes of Charles E. Tandy, you can *agree to, say no to, change, stop, or choose:*

- Doctors, nurses, social workers, health care providers; Hospitals, clinics, nursing homes, hospices, abodes; Medications, tests, treatments; Life support related issues; Surgery related issues; Comfort care and hospice care issues. *You may look at the medical records of Charles E. Tandy to help you make these decisions on behalf of the patient.*

Specific instructions regarding Life-Sustaining Treatment and Scope of Treatment:

- You will follow the guidelines that the patient (Charles E. Tandy) has provided.

Generic instructions as the Patient Advocate:

- You should always act with the patient's best interests and not your own interests.

- You will only start making decisions for the patient after 2 doctors agree that the patient is too sick to make his or her own decisions.

- You will not be able to make decisions that the patient would not usually be able to make.

- You don't have the power to stop a pregnant patient's treatment if it would cause her to die.

- You can make a decision to stop or not start treatments and allow the patient to die naturally if they have made it clear that you can make that decision.

- You cannot be paid for your role as a Patient Advocate but you can get paid back for the money you spend on the patient's medical expenses.

- You should help to protect the patient's rights as defined by law.

- You cannot make decisions that go against the patients' wishes regarding organ donation.

- The patient can remove you as Patient Advocate whenever they want.

- You can remove yourself as Patient Advocate whenever you want.

By signing, I am saying that I understand what this document says and that I will be the Patient Advocate for Charles E. Tandy.

{3rd Patient Advocate's Signature: Date: }

Name: ******
Address: ******
Telephone: ******

As the Patient Advocate (Surrogate Decision Maker)
– 4th Patient Advocate: ****** –

Based on the wishes of Charles E. Tandy, you can *agree to, say no to, change, stop, or choose:*

- Doctors, nurses, social workers, health care providers; Hospitals, clinics, nursing homes, hospices, abodes; Medications, tests, treatments; Life support related issues; Surgery related issues; Comfort care and hospice care issues. *You may look at the medical records of Charles E. Tandy to help you make these decisions on behalf of the patient.*

Specific instructions regarding Life-Sustaining Treatment and Scope of Treatment:

- You will follow the guidelines that the patient (Charles E. Tandy) has provided.

Generic instructions as the Patient Advocate:

- You should always act with the patient's best interests and not your own interests.

- You will only start making decisions for the patient after 2 doctors agree that the patient is too sick to make his or her own decisions.

- You will not be able to make decisions that the patient would not usually be able to make.

- You don't have the power to stop a pregnant patient's treatment if it would cause her to die.

- You can make a decision to stop or not start treatments and allow the patient to die naturally if they have made it clear that you can make that decision.

- 119 -

- You cannot be paid for your role as a Patient Advocate but you can get paid back for the money you spend on the patient's medical expenses.

- You should help to protect the patient's rights as defined by law.

- You cannot make decisions that go against the patients' wishes regarding organ donation.

- The patient can remove you as Patient Advocate whenever they want.

- You can remove yourself as Patient Advocate whenever you want.

By signing, I am saying that I understand what this document says and that I will be the Patient Advocate for Charles E. Tandy.

{4th Patient Advocate's Signature: _____ Date: _____ }
Name: ******
Address: ******
Telephone: ******

These sample documents and forms are designed to help cryonics counselors manage their responsibilities effectively and provide the best possible care for their clients. Feel free to adapt and expand these templates to suit your specific needs and circumstances.

Feel free to adjust or expand on this document to better fit the specific focus and style of your Guidebook!

YOUR NOTES HERE

www.ingramcontent.com/pod-product-compliance
Lightning Source LLC
Chambersburg PA
CBHW021342290326
41933CB00037B/426